T0293147

# PERCUTANEOUS CORONARY INTERVENTION

# PROCEDURES, MEDICAL USES AND ADVERSE EFFECTS

# CARDIOLOGY RESEARCH AND CLINICAL DEVELOPMENTS

Additional books in this series can be found on Nova's website under the Series tab.

Additional e-books in this series can be found on Nova's website under the e-book tab.

# PERCUTANEOUS CORONARY INTERVENTION

# PROCEDURES, MEDICAL USES AND ADVERSE EFFECTS

HUILI GAN

AND

YUJIE ZHOU

EDITORS

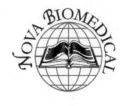

*New York*

Copyright © 2013 by Nova Science Publishers, Inc.

For permission to use material from this book please contact us:
Telephone 631-231-7269; Fax 631-231-8175
Web Site: http://www.novapublishers.com

### NOTICE TO THE READER

The Publisher has taken reasonable care in the preparation of this book, but makes no expressed or implied warranty of any kind and assumes no responsibility for any errors or omissions. No liability is assumed for incidental or consequential damages in connection with or arising out of information contained in this book. The Publisher shall not be liable for any special, consequential, or exemplary damages resulting, in whole or in part, from the readers' use of, or reliance upon, this material. Any parts of this book based on government reports are so indicated and copyright is claimed for those parts to the extent applicable to compilations of such works.

Independent verification should be sought for any data, advice or recommendations contained in this book. In addition, no responsibility is assumed by the publisher for any injury and/or damage to persons or property arising from any methods, products, instructions, ideas or otherwise contained in this publication.

This publication is designed to provide accurate and authoritative information with regard to the subject matter covered herein. It is sold with the clear understanding that the Publisher is not engaged in rendering legal or any other professional services. If legal or any other expert assistance is required, the services of a competent person should be sought. FROM A DECLARATION OF PARTICIPANTS JOINTLY ADOPTED BY A COMMITTEE OF THE AMERICAN BAR ASSOCIATION AND A COMMITTEE OF PUBLISHERS.

Additional color graphics may be available in the e-book version of this book.

**Library of Congress Cataloging-in-Publication Data**

Library of Congress Control Number: 2013939114

ISBN: 978-1-62618-962-1

*Published by Nova Science Publishers, Inc. † New York*

# Contents

# Preface

Cardiovascular disease is steadily increasing in developing countries and remains a major public health problem in developed countries, and is one of the most common causes of death. Among cardiovascular diseases, ACS comprises over 50% of deaths and the prevalence is also rising steadily. Since the September of 1977 when Dr. Gruentzig, the American physician, successfully completed the world's first case of percutaneous transluminal coronary angioplasty (PTCA), the percutaneous coronary intervention (PCI) has entered its third decade. In the past 30 years, PCI had gone through PTCA era, BMS era, and entered into the DES era. As an important part of the treatment of coronary heart disease, PCI technology not only improve the quality of life of the patient, expand their life expectancy, but also save a large number of lives. With the continuous development of new interventional devices, interventional techniques, ever evolving adjunctive pharmacotherapy, as well as the deepening understand to the pathophysiological mechanisms of different types of coronary heart disease, more importantly, evidence-based medicine adopted in the field of interventional cardiology, the PCI technology got its appropriate position in the overall strategy of coronary heart disease treatment.

Now, the percutaneous coronary intervention (PCI) is widely used to restore the blood flow to the stenosed coronary artery, and it has become the cornerstone of the treatment of ischemic heart disease. More than 1.2 million PCI procedures are performed annually in the United States, and it becomes also more and more popular in other countries and even in the developing countries. Recent advances in angioplasty equipment and technique have improved options for patients with smaller coronary and peripheral access arteries, and procedures through radial artery constitutes a much larger percentage of the overall percutaneous coronary interventions. In addition, the increased use of stents and adjunctive pharmacotherapy has also improved outcomes. percutaneous coronary intervention and adjunctive pharmacotherapy in reducing fatal and nonfatal ischemic complications in acute myocardial infarction and high-risk acute coronary syndromes have established tremendous benefits. With the creation and validation of new devices, new technologies and new adjuvant therapy, such great progress has been made in the field of coronary heart disease treatment; however, many problems and pitfalls remain unresolved, limiting further clinical application of PCI.

Percutaneous coronary intervention (PCI) is a field in rapid progression, over the last decade, knowledge in this field has grown consistently and significantly. The major disadvantage of percutaneous coronary intervention (PCI) in the treatment of patients with atherosclerotic coronary disease is the occurrence of restenosis and thrombus formation. To overcome these pitfalls, much effort has been made with an emphasis on the prevention of the restenosis. The purpose of our book *Percutaneous Coronary Intervention: Procedures, Medical Uses and Adverse Effects,* is to review what is known and not known about PCI, and to put these data be published in context with contemporary coronary intervention. This book summarized information gathered from recent literatures. A thorough and deep review of the literature was also conducted by our authors, some of whom are on the front lines of cutting-edge research or clinical practice. The chapter "Coronary Artery Lesion Assessment Techniques" detailed at different modalities that have been developed to fully identify flow-limiting lesions, including Intravascular Ultrasound (IVUS), and Optical Coherence Tomography (OCT); The chapter "Functional Coronary Magnetic Resonance Imaging" depicted at the advantages of functional coronary magnetic resonance imaging over X-ray coronary angiography and its usage in the clinical environment; The chapter "Inner catheter use for coronary angioplasty" introduced inner catheter that has been developed for difficult stent delivery cases; the chapter "Nucleic Acid Drugs to Prevent Restenosis after Coronary Intervention" descripted fully the effectiveness of an NF-B decoy ODN for preventing restenosis using experimental studies and clinical trials. The chapter: "Pharmacological Agents During Percutaneous Coronary Intervention" talked about evidence related to the various pharmacological agents available to clinicians during and after PCI. The last two chapters were to compare the PCI with CABG procedure in dealing with special subtype of coronary artery lesion, i.e. ostial right coronary lesion or left main coronary lesion, one of which compared the relative merits of PCI to CABG procedure in dealing with the ostial right coronary lesions, another chapter introduced the safeness of off-pump coronary artery bypass surgery in dealing Left main coronary artery lesion—in high volume cardiac surgery center.

I believe this book could provide useful and valuable information for the professionals in the field of cardiology and cardiac surgery and medical student; I also wish this book be conducive to the undertakings of the prevention and management of the cardiovascular disease, especially coronary heart disease.

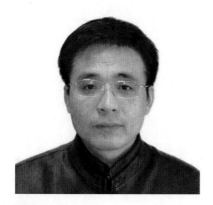

*Hui Li Gan*

Hui-Li Gan, MD, Ph.D
Professor of Cardiac Surgery
Department of Cardiac Surgery,
Beijing Anzhen Hospital, Capital Medical University,
Beijing Institute of Heart, Lung and Blood Vessel Diseases,
Beijing 100029, China

December 5, 2012 in Beijing

(Conflict of Interest Disclosures: The author (Hui-Li Gan) now serves as a local experienced surgeon in the phase III trials --the CHEST-1 and CHEST-2 study--on Riociguat, a novel drug that is currently in clinical development by Bayer Schering Pharma

Sources of Funding: This article was supported by a grant from National Natural Science Foundation of China (No. 81070041), and partly supported by grants from the Beijing Science and Technology Project (No.Z121107001012067) to Dr. Hui-Li Gan.

In: Percutaneous Coronary Intervention          ISBN: 978-1-62618-962-1
Editors: Huili Gan and Yujie Zhou     © 2013 Nova Science Publishers, Inc.

*Chapter I*

# Coronary Artery Lesion Assessment Techniques

*Haris Zafarullah, Kedar Sankholkar, Jay V. Doshi,*
*Wilbert S. Aronow\* and William Gotsis*
Cardiology Division, Westchester Medical Center
New York Medical College, Valhalla, NY, US

## Abstract

Understanding the clinical significance of an atherosclerotic plaque with its associated morbidity and mortality requires a multi-modal approach. Atherosclerosis is assessed invasively in the cardiac catheterization laboratory by coronary angiography. However, coronary angiography is somewhat limited by its two-dimensional imaging and its inability to assess remodeling. Therefore, it is not able to fully identify flow-limiting lesions.

Moreover, inter and intra-observer variability can contribute to inaccurate angiographic lesion assessment and evaluation, sometimes leading to intervention. To better assess the severity of coronary lesions, different modalities have been developed. These modalities include Intravascular Ultrasound (IVUS), Fractional Flow Reserve (FFR), and Optical Coherence Tomography (OCT). In this chapter, we will discuss

\* Tel: 914-493-5311; Fax: 914-235-6274; E-mail: wsaronow@aol.com.

the various applications of IVUS including pre and post intervention lesion assessment, the use of FFR as a vessel and lesion-specific stress test and its ability to assess the hemodynamic significance of a lesion, and finally the use of OCT as a higher resolution modality.

# Introduction

Atherosclerosis is assessed invasively in the cardiac catheterization laboratory by coronary angiography. However, coronary angiography is limited by its two-dimensional imaging and its inability to assess remodeling. Therefore, it is not able to fully identify flow-limiting lesions. To better assess the severity of coronary lesions, different modalities have been developed.

## Intravascular Ultrasound

Intravascular ultrasound (IVUS), a technology developed over two decades ago, has provided advances in our comprehension, evaluation and treatment of the atherosclerotic process.

There are two types of IVUS catheters:

1) Mechanical single-element rotating transducer
2) Solid-state electronic phased array transducer

Overall, they gain similar information regarding a lesion. The mechanical rotating transducer provides a smooth, incremental pullback and operates at higher ultrasound frequencies, thus providing greater resolution. The solid-state electronic transducer provides enhanced trackability and no non-uniform rotational distortion (NURD) artifact [1]. For spatial resolution with a 30-40MHz IVUS transducer, the typical resolution is 80-100 microns axially and 200-250 microns laterally.

## Pre-Intervention Lesion Assessment

Examples of angiographic findings exist that should prompt the interventionalist to utilize IVUS for further lesion investigation include intermediate lesions (40-70% angiographic stenosis) [2], left main (LM) disease, proximal or ostial disease, bifurcation stenosis, unusual morphology including aneurysms, calcification (Figure 1), thrombus, or times when there are discrepancies among the clinical case, angiographic findings, and other imaging modalities (Figure 2).

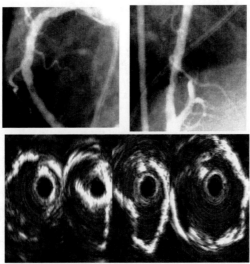

(with permission from Boston Scientific).

Figure 1. Unusual lesion morphology. A) Angiogram of hazy lesion; B) IVUS of same area depicting calcified plaque.

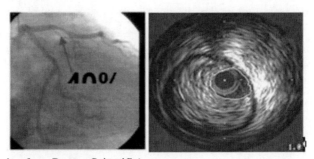

(with permission from Boston Scientific).

Figure 2. Discrepancies in clinical case resolved by IVUS. A 58-year-old male presented with unstable angina with anterior and inferior ECG changes upon exercise with no perfusion abnormalities on thallium. A) Angiogram revealing an intermediate lesion; B) IVUS of same lesion with 3.7mm$^2$ lumen cross-sectional area (CSA), or 95% stenosis.

**Table 1. Angiographic Plaque Characteristics Prompting IVUS Use**

| |
|---|
| Intermediate lesions severity (40-70% stenosis) |
| Lesion location (bifurcation, left main, ostium) |
| Hazy appearance |
| Aneurysms |
| Calcification |
| Thrombus |
| Discrepancy among imaging modalities |

In times where angiographic imaging falls short of providing optimal visualization of an arterial segment, IVUS proves particularly useful. Some examples include vessel tortuosity and overlapping vasculature.

## IVUS Protocol

The assessment of atherosclerotic plaque with IVUS involves determining plaque length (via motorized transducer pullback), volume, and content as well as the environment within which the plaque resides. Quantification of an atherosclerotic lesion begins with basic measurements of the surrounding vascular territory. These measurements involve identification of reference segments both proximal and distal to the lesion, the minimal lumen area (MLA) in between those two areas, and the external elastic membrane (EEM). After calculating the reference lumen area (RLA), or the areas proximal or distal to the stenosis, and the MLA in between those areas, one calculates the area stenosis and plaque burden (Figure 3):

*Area Stenosis*=(RLA – MLA)/ RLA X 100%
*Plaque Burden*=(EEM – Lumen) / EEM

An important factor in maintaining reproducibility of one's IVUS imaging is to document bifurcations within the lesion's vicinity. Once the basic measurements have been derived, plaque morphology can be assessed.

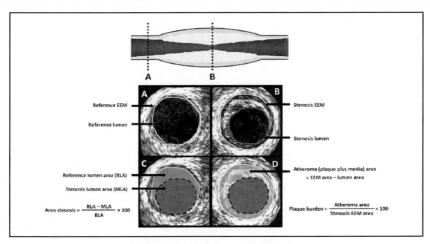

(Reference 1).

Figure 3. Basic IVUS measurements.

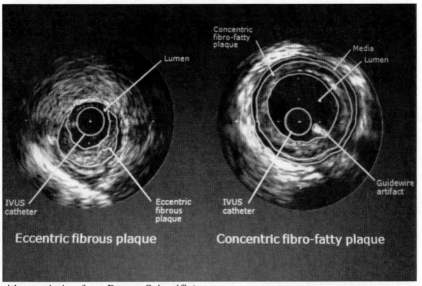

(with permission from Boston Scientific).

Figure 4. Plaque morphology. A) Eccentric fibrous plaque; B) Concentric fibro-fatty plaque.

IVUS can characterize several different types of plaque including soft, fibrous, calcified, or mixed [3].

Additionally, plaque length, volume, and eccentricity can be measured with IVUS (Figure 4).

# Clinical Applications of IVUS

## Predictor of Cardiovascular Outcomes

IVUS' ability for direct visualization of plaque characteristics allows identification of lesions that may contribute to cardiovascular morbidity and mortality.

Morphologic characteristics that are independent predictors of cardiovascular events include an MLA<4mm$^2$, a plaque burden of >70%, and thin-cap fibroatheroma (TCFA) [4].

## Left Main Disease

LM lesions have traditionally had the most angiographic inter-observer variability. In the Assessment of Intermediate Left Main Coronary Artery Lesions study (LITRO), an MLA > 6.0 mm$^2$ was prospectively identified to be a safe cut-off to defer revascularization of an angiographically intermediate LM lesion [5]. In patients who underwent elective percutaneous coronary intervention of the unprotected left main artery (ULM), there was a long-term mortality benefit of IVUS guided drug-eluting stent placement as compared to angiography only [6].

Recent studies have compared IVUS to fractional flow reserve (FFR) specifically in the LM and a suggested IVUS-calculated MLA that correlates with an FFR of <0.8 is 4.8mm$^2$ [7].

## Stent Apposition

Proper stent placement, expansion, and apposition are associated with lower event rates including in-stent restenosis and thrombosis [8]. IVUS is notably superior to angiography in achieving optimal stent expansion and apposition (Figure 5). Criteria have been validated for optimal stent deployment (Table 2).

**Table 2. IVUS Criteria for Optimal Stent Deployment (adapted from reference 1)**

| MUSIC Criteria | AVIO Criteria |
|---|---|
| Complete apposition of stent | Minimal post-stent area> 70% of the balloon cross-sectional area used to post-dilate the stent |
| Adequate stent expansion MSA $\geq$ 90% of an average reference lumen area or $\geq$ 100% of reference segment with the lowest area when the MSA is >9 mm$^2$ or MSA $\geq$ 80% of an average reference lumen area or $\geq$ 90% of reference segment with the lowest area when the MSA is >9 mm$^2$ | The noncompliant post-dilation balloon size selected according to the average of the maximum and minimum media-to-media diameter at the following points: 1. Distal in-stent segment 2. Proximal in-stent segment 3. In-stent of maximal narrowing |
| Symmetrical stent expansion Defined by minimum lumen diameter devide by maximum lumen diameter $\geq$ 0.7 | |

The criteria for optimal stent deployment used in the MUSIC (33) and AVIO (46) studies.

AVIO = Angiography Versus IVUS Optimization study; IVUS = intravascular ultrasound; MSA = minimal stent area; MUSIC = Multicenter Guided Stent Implantation in the Coronaries study.

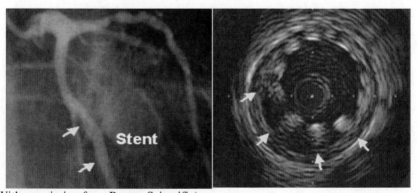

(With permission from Boston Scientific).

Figure 5. Stent apposition. A) Angiographic view of stent in coronary artery appearing well apposed; B) Same vessel with stent showing clear mal-apposition.

## Edge Dissection

Edge dissection has a prevalence of approximately 10% and is often angiographically silent [1]. Because of the associated high incidence of post-stent thrombosis and cardiovascular complications, edge dissections mandate further investigation and possible intervention (Figure 8).

## Stent Fracture

Stent fracture can be hard to identify on coronary angiography and manifests as haziness. However, IVUS has been shown to be helpful in identifying stent fracture [9].

## In-Stent Restenosis

IVUS can be utilized to identify stent under-deployment which is one of the risk factors of in-stent restenosis [10]. Studies have shown that in IVUS-guided bare metal stent implantation, post-angioplasty MLD>6.0 results in low restenosis rates comparable to drug-eluting stents [11].

## Identification of Vulnerable Plaque

Virtual Histology (VH) utilizes spectral analysis to color-code various histological characteristics of a plaque (Figure 6). In the VIVA (VH-IVUS in Vulnerable Atherosclerosis) Study, patients who were found to have thin-cap fibroatheroma by VH-IVUS had higher levels of non-restenotic major adverse cardiovascular events (MACE) [12]. Thus VH-IVUS may be able to identify vulnerable plaques with the potential to cause myocardial infarction [4]. In conclusion, IVUS has a role in morphological lesion assessment and can assist in optimal stent deployment to prevent adverse cardiovascular outcomes.

## Fractional Flow Reserve

Fractional flow reserve (FFR) is an invasive assessment of coronary lesions.

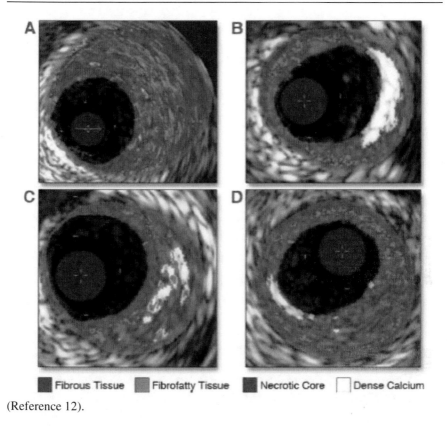

Fibrous Tissue    Fibrofatty Tissue    Necrotic Core    Dense Calcium

(Reference 12).

Figure 6. Plaque classification by VH-IVUS. A) Pathologic intimal thickening; B) fibrocalcific plaque; C) thick-cap fibroatheroma; D) thin-cap fibroatheroma (TCFA).

It has been well validated and is shown to correlate with non-invasive stress testing [13, 14]. FFR is the maximum myocardial blood flow in the presence of a stenosis divided by normal maximum blood flow. It is derived by the following calculation:

FFR =Maximum myocardial blood flow in the presence of a stenosis/normal maximum blood flow.

## Protocol for FFR

The coronary artery is engaged with a guide catheter and anti-coagulation is given with heparin or bivaluridin. A 0.14 pressure wire is placed proximally before the lesion and proximal pressure measurements are recorded.

The lesion is then crossed and hyperemia is achieved. Pressure measurements are taken while the patient is in a hyperemic state. The distal pressure is divided by the proximal pressure and results in a decimal number (or Fractional Flow Reserve number).

## Choice of Hyperemic Stimuli

Maximal hyperemia can be achieved by different agents and either via intravenous or Intracoronary administration. The agents used for inducing hyperemia are adenosine, papaverine, and dipyridamole.

Adenosine is the preferred agent for inducing hyperemia because of its short action. The intravenous route is preferred as it allows a steady state of infusion.

## FFR Threshold for Ischemia

The FFR values are divided into three categories:

- Less than 0.75 in which the lesion is flow-limiting and intervention is indicated.
- Values above 0.80 suggest that the lesion can be safely deferred.
- Between 0.75 – 0.80, which is in the intermediate area.

# Clinical Applications of FFR

## Intermediate Angiographic Lesions

Coronary stenosis which is angiographically intermediate (between 40-70%) can be further assessed by FFR. In the Deferral Versus Performance of PTCA in Patients Without Documented Ischemia (DEFER) trial, lesions with FFR values more than 0.75 were assigned to optimal medical therapy, and FFR values less than 0.75 underwent percutaneous coronary intervention (PCI) [15].

In the five-year follow-up, survival was equal in both groups, and patients who had FFR values greater than 0.75 had a less than 1% risk of death or myocardial infarction.

## Multivessel Coronary Artery Disease

FFR can be used to identify flow-limiting hemodynamic lesions in angiographically appearing significant multi vessel coronary artery disease (CAD). Studies have shown that by using FFR, there are less flow-limiting lesions and the non hemodynamically significant lesions can be managed with medical therapy with no adverse outcomes [16].

## Microvascular Disease

Patients with microvascular disease can have angiographically significant lesions. If the microvasular disease is significant, then intervening on the vessel will not improve flow [17, 18]. Therefore FFR can guide therapy in patients with significant microvascular disease and epicardial stenosis.

## Left Main Disease

Left main disease can be hard to quantify angiographically. IVUS has been studied and is well validated in left main disease. FFR has also been studied in left main disease. In a 3-year follow-up, FFR guidance with values greater than 0.75 were assigned to optimal medical therapy and there was no adverse cardiovascular outcomes [19, 20]

## Serial Lesions

For serial stenosis, pull back FFR is done to assess the severity of individual lesions. [21]. The wire is placed distal to the last lesion, and hyperemia is induced. Once FFR becomes significant, a gradual pullback is done with continuous recording.

## Bifurcations and Jailed Side Branches

When a stent is placed across a bifurcation lesion, there is plaque shift across the side branch, and the side branch may look worse. Angiography is unable to assess the lesion severity. FFR has been studied in post stenting side branches and if the lesion is not significant by FFR and it was managed medically, there were no long-term adverse outcomes [22].

## FFR in Acute Coronary Syndromes

FFR has not been studied in ST-elevation myocardial infarction (STEMI) patients as there is concern that the values will be misleading because of microvasculature changes [23]. In the Fractional Flow Reserve Versus Angiography for Multivessel Evaluation (FAME) trial, FFR was done in unstable angina and non –STEMI patients and was safe [24].

## FFR in Post STEMI Patients

Patients with STEMI who undergo revascularization of the culprit lesion may have other lesions. It is recommended that those lesions should not be intervened at the time of STEMI. FFR is a helpful technology to assess the hemodynamic severity of the non-culprit lesions [25].

## Previous Myocardial Infarction

An infarcted myocardium will require less blood flow as compared to a normal myocardium. Therefore, the FFR value in infarcted myocardium will be non-significant [26].

## Post PCI Management

FFR has been studied in immediately post PCI patients, and values of more than 0.90 correlate with better long-term outcomes [27].

## FFR in Stable CAD with Optimal Medical Management

In patients with stable CAD who are on optimal medical management, FFR can guide management of hemodynamically significant lesions.

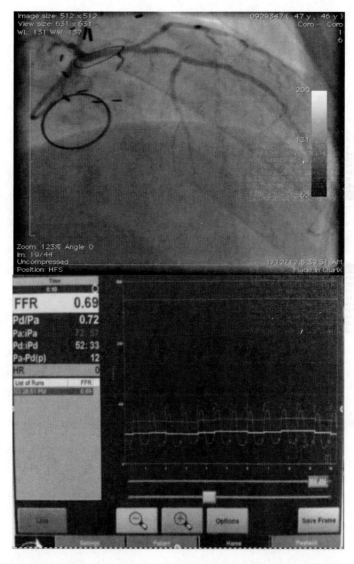

Figure 7. Patient with Canadian Cardiovascular Society Class III who underwent coronary angiography with a moderate lesion in left anterior descending (LAD) coronary artery, and FFR was significant at 0.69.

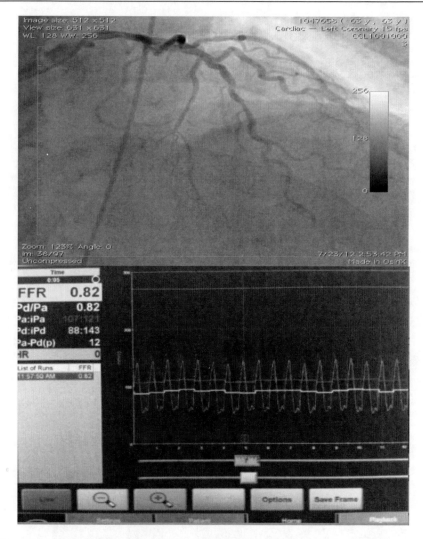

Figure 8. Patient with atypical chest discomfort who underwent coronary angiogram with a moderate lesion in LAD, and FFR was non-significant at 0.82.

In a recent study patients with stable CAD who had a hemodynamically significant lesion by FFR and underwent PCI had less frequent admissions for angina. [28] It should be noted that there was no difference in all-cause cardiovascular mortality.

In conclusion, FFR is a vessel and lesion-specific stress test within the cardiac catheterization laboratory with a high accuracy and offers significant savings and clinical benefit to the patient.

# Optical Coherence Tomography (OCT)

## Methodology

Intravascular optical coherence tomography (OCT) is an intravascular imaging modality that uses the reflection and scattering of light to create arterial wall imaging. Compared to other imaging modalities, OCT offers a much better image resolution and localization of image origin, reaching 10-20 microns [29]. OCT can use two different technologies to obtain images: time-domain and frequency domain. The currently available method is the frequency domain, which records the backscattering of light from the vessel wall. Although technology is improving, currently frequency-domain OCT achieves an axial resolution of 10-15 micrometers, lateral resolution of 40-90 micrometers and tissue penetration of 2-3.5 mm. [29]

Limitations of OCT include penetration depth, inability to image through a blood field, and difficulty in imaging proximal target sites, particularly for ostial left main and right coronary artery lesions.

# Clinical Applications of OCT

## Use for Assessment of Coronary Lesions

Studies have shown that OCT has improved sensitivity than IVUS in identifying these lesions. In one study by Prati et al., OCT confirmed the presence of complicated plaques in 61% of the patients; IVUS underdiagnosed these patients with only 48% identified to have complicated plaques [30]. OCT provides an excellent modality to differentiate between the lumen and arterial layers, allowing clear differentiation between the intima and media.

As in IVUS, OCT is useful in quantifying lesion severity better than coronary angiography alone. Unlike IVUS, OCT can identify plaque ulceration and thrombus formation.

## Stenting and the Role of OCT

OCT , due to its ability to obtain high resolution imaging of the vessel-tissue interface, can be used to look at stent apposition after deployment.

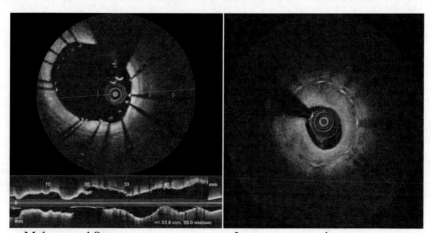

Malapposed Struts                          In-stent restenosis
(with permission from Saint Jude Medical).

Figure 9. OCT of malapposed struts and in-stent restenosis.

OCT can identify stent malapposition, uneven stent strut distribution and intrastent small thrombotic formations, more readily as compared to IVUS, and further decrease rates of drug-eluting stents (DES) failure due to restenosis and stent thrombosis [31]. Figure 9 depicts malapposed struts and in-stent restenosis.

# Conclusion

The appropriate treatment for any specific patient takes into account multiple factors. A systematic approach useful in clinical scenarios includes the use of FFR as a determining methodology for appropriateness for intervention if no noninvasive testing was performed. IVUS assessment should be performed pre and post intervention for optimal treatment strategy. OCT may also be used instead of IVUS, but is less widely used at this time.

# References

[1]    McDaniel M. C, Eshtehardi P, Sawaya F. J, et al. Contemporary clinical applications of coronary intravascular ultrasound. *JACC Cardiovasc. Interv.* 2011; 4: 1155-1167.

[2]   Briguori C, Anzuini A, Airoldi F, et al. Intravascular ultrasound criteria for the assessment of the functional significance of intermediate coronary artery stenoses and comparison with fractional flow reserve. *Am. J. Cardiol.* 2001; 87: 136-141.

[3]   Garcia-Garcia H. M, Costa M. A, Serruys P. W. Imaging of coronary atherosclerosis: intravascular ultrasound. *Eur. Heart J.* 2010; 31: 2456-2469.

[4]   Stone G. W, Maehara A, Lansky A. J, et al. A prospective natural-history study of coronary atherosclerosis. *N. Engl. J. Med.* 2011; 364: 226-235.

[5]   de la Torre Hernandez J. M, Hernández Hernandez F, Alfonso F, et al. Prospective Application of Pre-Defined Intravascular Ultrasound Criteria for Assessment of Intermediate Left Main Coronary Artery Lesions: Results From the Multicenter LITRO Study. *J. Am. Coll. Cardiol.* 2011; 58:351-358.

[6]   Park, S. J, Kim Y. H, Park D. W et al. Impact of intravascular ultrasound guidance on long-term mortality in stenting for unprotected left main coronary artery stenosis." *Circulation Cardiovasc. Interv.* 2009; 2: 167-177.

[7]   Kang, S. J, Lee J. Y, Ahn J. M, et al. Intravascular ultrasound-derived predictors for fractional flow reserve in intermediate left main disease *JACC Cardiovasc. Interv.* 2011 ;4: 1168-1174.

[8]   Yoon, HJ, Hur SH. Optimization of stent deployment by intravascular ultrasound. Korean *J. Intern. Med.* 2012; 27: 30-38.

[9]   Fang H. Y, Bhasin A, Youssef A, et al. Intravascular ultrasound (IVUS) guided fixation of an accidentally crushed coronary stent. *Int. Heart J.* 2008; 49: 621-627.

[10]  Sbruzzi G, Quadros A. S, Ribeiro R. A, et al. Intracoronary ultrasound-guided stenting improves outcomes: a meta-analysis of randomized trials. *Arq. Bras. Cardiol.* 2012; 98: 35-44.

[11]  de Feyter P. J, Kay P, Disco C, Serruys P. W. Reference chart derived from post-stent-implantation intravascular ultrasound predictors of 6-month expected restenosis on quantitative coronary angiography. *Circulation* 1999; 100: 1777-1783.

[12]  Calvert P. A, Obaid D. R, O'Sullivan M, et al. Association between IVUS findings and adverse outcomes in patients with coronary artery disease: the VIVA (VH-IVUS in Vulnerable Atherosclerosis) Study. *JACC Cardiovasc. Imaging.* 2011; 4: 894-901.

[13]  Pijls N. H, De Bruyne B, Peels K, et al. Measurement of fractional flow reserve to assess the functional severity of coronary-artery stenoses. *N. Engl. J. Med.* 1996;334:1703-1708.

[14]  Bech G. J. W, De Bruyne B, Pijls N. H. J, et al. Fractional Flow Reserve to Determine the Appropriateness of Angioplasty in Moderate Coronary Stenosis, A Randomized Trial. *Circulation* 2001:103:2928-2934.

[15]  Pijls N. H, van Schaardenburgh P, Manoharan G, et al. Percutaneous coronary intervention of functionally nonsignificant stenosis: 5-year follow-up of the DEFER Study. *J. Am. Coll. Cardiol.* 2007; 49: 2105-11.

[16]  Botman K. J, Pijls N. H, Bech J. W, et al. Percutaneous coronary intervention or bypass surgery in multivessel disease? A tailored approach based on coronary pressure measurement. *Catheter Cardiovasc. Interv.* 2004; 63:184-91.

[17]  De Bruyne B, Sarma J. Fractional Flow Reserve: A Review. *Heart* 2008; 94:949-959.

[18]  Pijls H, FearonW. F, Tonino P. A. et al. Fractional Flow Reserve versus Angiography for Guiding Percutaneous Coronary Intervention. *N. Eng. J. Med.* 2009; 3:213-224.

[19]  Bech G. J, Droste H, Pijls N. H, et al. Value of fractional flow reserve in making decisions about bypass surgery for equivocal left main coronary artery disease. *Heart* 2001; 86:547-52.

[20]  Lindstaedt M, Yazar A, Germing A, et al. Clinical outcome in patients with intermediate or equivocal left main coronary artery disease after deferral of surgical revascularization on the basis of fractional flow reserve measurements. *Am. Heart J.* 2006;15:156.e1-9.

[21]  Pijls N. H., De Bruyne B, Bech G. J., et al. Coronary pressure measurement to assess the hemodynamic significance of serial stenoses within one coronary artery: validation in humans. *Circulation* 2000; 102:2371-7.

[22]  Koo B. K., Park K. W., Kang H. J., et al. Physiological evaluation of the provisional side branch intervention strategy for bifurcation lesions using fractional flow reserve. *Eur. Heart J.* 2008; 29:726-732.

[23]  Uren N. G., Crake T, Lefroy D. C., et al. Reduced coronary vasodilator function in infarcted and normal myocardium after myocardial infarction.*N. Engl. J. Med.* 1994; 331: 222-227.

[24]  Sels J. M., Tonino P. L., Siebert U, et al. Fractional Flow Reserve in Unstable Angina and Non–ST-Segment Elevation Myocardial Infarction: Experience from the FAME (Fractional flow reserve versus Angiography

for Multivessel Evaluation) Study. *J. Am. Coll. Cardiol. Intv.* 2011; 4: 1183-1189.

[25] Ntalianis A, Sels J, Davidavicius G, et al. Fractional Flow Reserve for the Assessment of Nonculprit Coronary Artery Stenoses in Patients With Acute Myocardial Infarction. *J. Am. Coll. Cardiol. Intv.* 2010; 3:1274-1281.

[26] De Bruyne B, Pijls N. H., Bartunek J, et al. Fractional flow reserve in patients with prior myocardial infarction. *Circulation* 2001; 104:157-62.

[27] Pijls N. H. J., Klauss V, Siebert U, et al. Coronary pressure measurement after stenting predicts adverse events at follow-up: A multicenter registry. *Circulation* 2002; 105: 2950-2954.

[28] De Bruyne B, Pijls N, Kalesan B, et al. Fractional flow reserve-guided PCI versus medical therapy in stable coronary disease. *N. Engl. J. Med.* 2012; 367: 991-1001.

[29] Prati F, Regar E, Mintz G. S., et al. Expert review document on methodology, terminology, and clinical applications of optical coherence tomography: physical principles, methodology of image acquisition, and clinical application for assessment of coronary arteries and atherosclerosis. *Eur. Heart J.* 2010; 31: 401-415.

[30] Prati F, Imola F. Stent Sizing and Deployment with Optical Coherence Tomography Guidance. *Interventional Cardiology* 2009; 4:31-33.

[31] Roy P, Steinberg D. H., Sushinsky S. I., et al. The potential clinical utility of intravascular ultrasound guidance in patients undergoing percutaneous coronary intervention with drug-eluting stents. *Eur. Heart J.* 2008; 29: 1851-7.

In: Percutaneous Coronary Intervention          ISBN: 978-1-62618-962-1
Editors: Huili Gan and Yujie Zhou          © 2013 Nova Science Publishers, Inc.

*Chapter II*

# Functional Coronary Magnetic Resonance Imaging

## *Sebastian Kelle*

Department of Internal Medicine/Cardiology,
Deutsches Herzzentrum Berlin, Germany

## Abstract

Coronary magnetic resonance imaging is a powerful non-invasive technique for the combined assessment of coronary artery anatomy and function. In the present review article, challenges in coronary artery imaging are discussed and results obtained in both healthy volunteers and patients with cardiovascular disease are presented. This includes an overview of coronary artery vessel lumen and wall imaging, new and specific contrast agents, molecular targeted imaging, permeability of the coronary vessel wall, high-field imaging, imaging(measurement of coronary distensibility and endothelial function and interventional coronary magnetic resonance imaging.

## Introduction

Coronary artery disease (CAD) remains the leading cause of death for men and women worldwide. X-ray coronary angiography, the current gold standard to diagnose CAD, is able to identify in vivo coronary vessel lumen stenosis but offers only limited information about the coronary artery vessel wall. The whole invasive procedure has the risk of complications and involves radiation exposure and the use of iodinated contrast agents [1, 2]. In addition, dependent on the pre-test probability of CAD, between 30% and up to 70% of patients who undergo invasive X-ray coronary angiography are found to have no significant coronary artery lumen stenosis [3].

Coronary magnetic resonance imaging (MRI) offers several advantages over X-ray coronary angiography. It is a non-invasive method with a relatively high spatial resolution and high soft-tissue contrast and has the ability to generate images in any three-dimensional plane without the need for ionizing radiation. Other advantages of coronary MRI are the possibility for repeated measurements and the ability to assess cardiac anatomy, function and viability simultaneously in a single examination [4].

## Coronary Artery Lumen Imaging

For adequate visualization of the coronary arteries, a high contrast between the coronary lumen and the surrounding tissue is crucial [4, 5].

There are only two multi-center trials of magnetic resonance coronary angiography (MRCA) to date. The first clearly demonstrated a high sensitivity, specificity (85%) and negative predictive value (100%) for the identification of left main stem or multi-vessel coronary artery disease [6]. In a subsequent single center study the use of a whole-heart technique to cover the entire coronary artery tree (similar to multi-slice computed tomography) was investigated [7].

In that study, a sensitivity of 82% and a specificity of 90% were obtained for the identification of significant CAD when compared to invasive X-ray coronary angiography [4, 7]. In addition, in a second multicenter trial using whole-heart coverage and no contrast agent at 3.0 Tesla a high sensitivity and specificity in general for the detection of CAD were reported [8]. However, the reported findings did not lead to routine clinical use of MRCA in symptomatic patients suspected of having hemodynamically significant CAD [6] (Figure 1).

A recent report directly compared the diagnostic accuracy of MRI and MSCT for the detection of CAD using 3.0-T MRI and 64-slice dual-source CT. In the patient-based analysis MRI and CT angiography showed similar diagnostic accuracy of 83% (95% confidence interval [CI]: 75 to 87) versus 87% (95% CI: 80 to 92), p = 0.38.

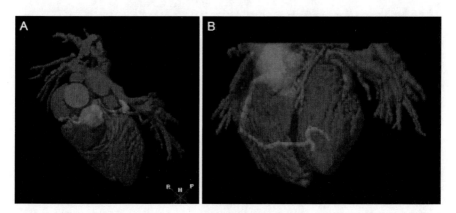

Figure 1. Volume-rendering method demonstrates three-dimensional view of left anterior descending artery (LAD) and right coronary artery (RCA).

The authors concluded that 32-channel 3.0-T MRI and 64-slice CT angiography similarly identify significant coronary stenosis in patients with suspected or known coronary artery disease scheduled for elective coronary angiography. However, CT angiography showed a favorable trend toward higher diagnostic performance [9]. Recently, the first study to determine whether whole-heart coronary magnetic resonance angiography (CMRA) can predict cardiac events in patients with suspected coronary artery disease has been reported. During a median follow-up of 25 months Cox regression analysis showed that presence of significant stenosis in CMRA was associated with a >20-fold hazard increase for all cardiac events (hazard ratio: 20.78; 95% confidence interval: 2.65 to 162.70; p = 0.001). The authors concluded that whole-heart CMRA was useful for predicting the future risk for cardiac events in patients with suspected coronary artery disease [10].

# Coronary Vessel Wall Imaging

The rupture of a high-risk atherosclerotic plaque may result in myocardial infarction and/or sudden cardiac death [11]. Identification of these plaques could lead to alterations in systemic (pharmacological) therapies and possibly guide local (interventional) therapies in patients at very high risk [11, 12].

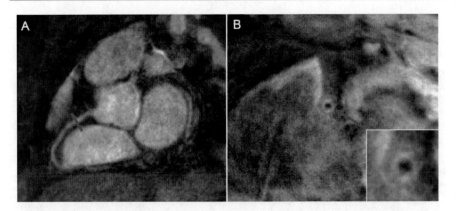

Figure 2. (A) Three-dimensional reformatted coronary MRI of the proximal RCA in asubject without coronary luminal stenosis but with long-standing type 2 diabetes. The corresponding three-dimensional black-blood vessel wall scan (B) shows no CMRI evidence of atherosclerotic plaque; however there is an increased atherosclerotic plaque burden.

Today, with clinical MRI scanners, the spatial resolution is too low to accurately characterize coronary plaque components. However, early studies demonstrated that coronary vessel wall thickness can be quantified non-invasively using "black-blood" MRI [13, 14].

MRI has also been demonstrated to be an appropriate non-invasive tool for the quantification of 'Glagov'-type [15] positive arterial remodelling [16]. A recent study in patients with type 1 diabetes demonstrated the ability of coronary MRI to visualize different stages of diabetes by measuring coronary vessel wall thickness [4, 17] (Figure 2).

In a further recent study, the prevalence, quality, and extent of coronary atherosclerosis in a group of healthy subjects compared to patients with confirmed CAD has been evaluated.

The authors found that, in this cohort of middle-aged individuals, both patients with stable angina and angiographically proven coronary artery disease as well as age-matched asymptomatic subjects exhibited coronary vessel wall thickening detectable with MR coronary vessel wall imaging. Maximum and mean wall thicknesses were significantly higher in patients. The vast majority of asymptomatic subjects had either positive remodeling without luminal narrowing or non-significant stenosis [18].

# Coronary Vessel Wall
# Delayed Enhancement

Late gadolinium enhancement (LGE) of the vascular (arterial) wall is a very promising method for evaluating carotid and aortic plaque and inflammatory vasculopathies [19-22].

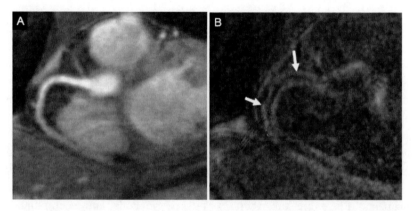

Figure 3. (A)Detection of coronary artery plaque enhancement. The RCA is demonstrated by three-dimensional reformatted coronary MRI. (B) Inversion recovery coronary MRI around 50 minutes after gadolinium application demonstrates diffuse enhancement of the RCA wall (white arrows).

In first human LGE studies of the coronary artery wall the potential for coronary artery plaque visualization and characterization using a T1-weighted coronary MRI technique has been demonstrated [23, 24]. Our group was able to achieve further improvement of the technique by using higher spatial resolution at higher field strengths (3.0-T MRI) and to evaluate the optimal time-point for implementation of this technique in clinical routine [25] (Figure 3). The findings of others and our study lead to the conclusion that LGE of the coronary vascular wall might be associated with increased vascular permeability (as may occur with inflammation) or with an increased distribution volume (as with fibrosis and neovascularization) in the altered coronary vessel wall [4]. In a recent study we evaluated coronary LGE in patients with chronic CAD compared to patients with Takayasu's arteritis (TA). We found that LGE of the coronary artery wall seems to be common in patients with TA and similarly pronounced as in CAD patients. However, the observed coronary LGE seems to be rather unspecific, and differentiation between coronary vessel wall fibrosis and inflammation remains unclear [26].

# Molecular Targeted Imaging

The development of contrast agents that offer the differentiation of specific plaque components seems to be very promising. However, molecular contrast agents targeted to fibrin, macrophages or high-density lipoprotein (HDL) have so far been tested only at the preclinical level [27-29]. Recent studies have demonstrated that vascular MRI using the fibrin-targeted contrast agent EP-2104R allows selective visualization of human clot material in a model of coronary thrombosis in swine [30] and of thrombi in the arterial vasculature and the ventricular chambers in humans [4, 31]. Macrophages are key inflammatory cells in atherosclerosis [12]. In a recently published animal study, areas of macrophage-rich plaques were highlighted and the magnitude of enhancement was significantly related to the histologically confirmed number of macrophages [32]. Additionally, to detect inflammatory areas, contrast agents that infiltrate inmunocompetent cells have been used, allowing these cells to be tracked and, as a consequence, enabling detection and characterization of inflammatory regions. Perfluorocarbons (PFCs), which contain a high concentration of $^{19}$F atoms, have been used in animal experiments. PFCs are taken up by phagocytic cells and accumulate in inflammatory regions, offering the possibility of detecting inflammation and potentially of monitoring treatment [33].

# Coronary Endothelial Function

Endothelial-dependent coronary artery vasomotor reactivity is an important indicator of vascular function and might be able to predict cardiovascular events [34]. Significant changes in coronary artery cross-sectional area and flow velocity occur in direct response to endothelial-dependent stressors (e.g. isometric handgrip or cold-pressure testing) and these can be detected by MRI methods [35]. In a recent study we tested two hypotheses: first, that coronary endothelial function can be measured noninvasively and abnormal function detected using clinical 3.0-T MRI; and, second, that the extent of local coronary CAD in a given patient is related to the degree of local abnormal coronary endothelial function. We found endothelial-dependent coronary artery dilation and increased blood flow in healthy subjects, and their absence in CAD patients. Local coronary endothelial function differed between severely and mildly diseased arteries in a given CAD patient. Therefore, this novel, safe method may offer new insights regarding the importance of local coronary endothelial function and improved risk stratification in patients at risk for and with known CAD [36] (Figure 4). In a further extension of our study we tested the hypothesis that abnormal coronary endothelial function is related to measures of early atherosclerosis such as increased coronary wall thickness. We found that there was an inverse relationship between coronary endothelial function and local coronary wall thickness in patients with coronary artery disease, but not in healthy adults. These findings demonstrated that local endothelial-dependent functional changes are related to the extent of early anatomic atherosclerosis in mildly diseased arteries. We concluded that this combined MRI approach enables the anatomic and functional investigation of early coronary disease [37].

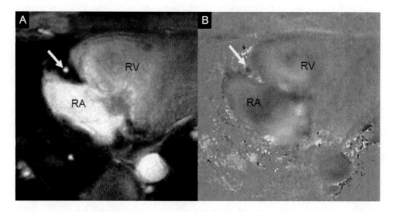

Figure 4. (A) A cross-sectional magnetic resonance angiography view from a healthy adult subject perpendicular to the RCA (white arrow) ( RA = right atrium; RV = right ventricle). (B). Flow velocity encoded MRI phase image of the RCA The signal intensity is proportional to flow velocity, with a black signal indicating high velocity down through the imaging plane (white arrow).

# Intravascular MR Imaging

Intravascular MRI with active internal probes offers high sensitivity to pathological features without ionizing radiation or the limited luminal views of conventional X-rays but has been unable to provide a high-speed, high-resolution, endoscopic view. In a recently published study, real-time MRI endoscopy was introduced for performing MRI from a viewpoint intrinsically locked to a miniature active, internal transmitter-receiver in a clinical 3.0-T MRI scanner. The authors describe how real-time MRI endoscopy at up to 2 frames/s was able to depict vascular wall morphological features, atherosclerosis, and calcification at 80 to 300 μm resolution during probe advancement through diseased human iliac artery specimens and atherosclerotic rabbit aortas in vivo. The reported findings offer the potential for fast, minimally invasive, transluminal, high-resolution imaging of vascular disease on a common clinical platform suitable for evaluating and targeting atherosclerosis in both experimental and clinical settings [38].

# Conclusion

Coronary magnetic resonance imaging is a powerful non-invasive technique for the combined assessment of coronary artery anatomy and function. The development of new and specific contrast agents and continued innovation in MRI methods will lead to further progress being made towards the non-invasive and comprehensive assessment of coronary atherosclerotic disease [4].

# Acknowledgments

The author would like to thank Anne Gale of the Deutsches Herzzentrum Berlin for expert assistance in preparation of the manuscript.

# References

[1] Davidson CJ, Mark DB, Pieper KS, et al. Thrombotic and cardiovascular complications related to nonionic contrast media during cardiac catheterization: analysis of 8,517 patients. *Am. J. Cardiol.*, 1990;65: 1481-4.
[2] Omran H, Schmidt H, Hackenbroch M, et al. Silent and apparent cerebral embolism after retrograde catheterisation of the aortic valve in valvular stenosis: a prospective, randomised study. *Lancet,* 2003;361: 1241-6.

[3]   Patel MR, Peterson ED, Dai D, et al. Low diagnostic yield of elective coronary angiography. *N. Engl. J. Med.,* 2010;362:886-95.

[4]   Kelle S, Weiss RG, Stuber M. Coronary MR imaging: lumen and wall. *Magn. Reson. Imaging Clin. N Am.,* 2009;17:145-58.

[5]   Stuber M, Weiss RG. Coronary magnetic resonance angiography. *J. Magn. Reson. Imaging.,* 2007;26:219-34.

[6]   Kim WY, Danias PG, Stuber M, et al. Coronary magnetic resonance angiography for the detection of coronary stenoses. *N. Engl. J. Med.,* 2001;345:1863-9.

[7]   Sakuma H, Ichikawa Y, Chino S, Hirano T, Makino K, Takeda K. Detection of coronary artery stenosis with whole-heart coronary magnetic resonance angiography. *J. Am. Coll. Cardiol.,* 2006;48:1946-50.

[8]   Kato S, Kitagawa K, Ishida N, et al. Assessment of Coronary Artery Disease Using Magnetic Resonance Coronary AngiographyA National Multicenter Trial. *Journal of the American College of Cardiology,* 2010;56:983-991.

[9]   Hamdan A, Asbach P, Wellnhofer E, et al. A prospective study for comparison of MR and CT imaging for detection of coronary artery stenosis. *JACC Cardiovasc Imaging,* 2011;4:50-61.

[10]  Yoon YE, Kitagawa K, Kato S, et al. Prognostic Value of Coronary Magnetic Resonance Angiography for Prediction of Cardiac Events in Patients With Suspected Coronary Artery Disease. *Journal of the American College of Cardiology, 2012*;60:2316-2322.

[11]  Naghavi M, Libby P, Falk E, et al. From vulnerable plaque to vulnerable patient: a call for new definitions and risk assessment strategies: Part I. *Circulation,* 2003;108:1664-72.

[12]  Libby P. Inflammation in atherosclerosis. *Nature,* 2002;420:868-74.

[13]  Fayad ZA, Fuster V, Fallon JT, et al. Noninvasive in vivo human coronary artery lumen and wall imaging using black-blood magnetic resonance imaging. *Circulation,* 2000;102:506-10.

[14]  Edelman RR, Chien D, Kim D. Fast selective black blood MR imaging. *Radiology,* 1991;181:655-60.

[15]  Glagov S, Weisenberg E, Zarins CK, Stankunavicius R, Kolettis GJ. Compensatory enlargement of human atherosclerotic coronary arteries. *N. Engl. J. Med.,* 1987;316:1371-5.

[16]  Kim WY, Stuber M, Bornert P, Kissinger KV, Manning WJ, Botnar RM. Three-dimensional black-blood cardiac magnetic resonance coronary vessel wall imaging detects positive arterial remodeling in

patients with nonsignificant coronary artery disease. *Circulation,* 2002;106:296-9.

[17]   Kim WY, Astrup AS, Stuber M, et al. Subclinical coronary and aortic atherosclerosis detected by magnetic resonance imaging in type 1 diabetes with and without diabetic nephropathy. *Circulation,* 2007;115:228-35.

[18]   Gerretsen SC, Kooi ME, Kessels AG, et al. Visualization of coronary wall atherosclerosis in asymptomatic subjects and patients with coronary artery disease using magnetic resonance imaging. *PLoS One,* 2010;5.

[19]   Desai MY, Lai S, Barmet C, Weiss RG, Stuber M. Reproducibility of 3D free-breathing magnetic resonance coronary vessel wall imaging. *Eur. Heart J.,* 2005;26:2320-4.

[20]   Yuan C, Kerwin WS, Ferguson MS, et al. Contrast-enhanced high resolution MRI for atherosclerotic carotid artery tissue characterization. *J. Magn. Reson. Imaging.,* 2002;15:62-7.

[21]   Cai J, Hatsukami TS, Ferguson MS, et al. In vivo quantitative measurement of intact fibrous cap and lipid-rich necrotic core size in atherosclerotic carotid plaque: comparison of high-resolution, contrast-enhanced magnetic resonance imaging and histology. *Circulation,* 2005;112:3437-44.

[22]   Wasserman BA, Smith WI, Trout HH, 3rd, Cannon RO, 3rd, Balaban RS, Arai AE. Carotid artery atherosclerosis: in vivo morphologic characterization with gadolinium-enhanced double-oblique MR imaging initial results. *Radiology,* 2002;223:566-73.

[23]   Maintz D, Ozgun M, Hoffmeier A, et al. Selective coronary artery plaque visualization and differentiation by contrast-enhanced inversion prepared MRI. *Eur. Heart J.,* 2006;27:1732-6.

[24]   Yeon SB, Sabir A, Clouse M, et al. Delayed-enhancement cardiovascular magnetic resonance coronary artery wall imaging: comparison with multislice computed tomography and quantitative coronary angiography. *J. Am. Coll. Cardiol.,* 2007;50:441-7.

[25]   Kelle S, Schlendorf K, Hirsch GA, et al. Gadolinium Enhanced MR Coronary Vessel Wall Imaging at 3.0 Tesla. *Cardiol. Res. Pract.,* 2009;2010:856418.

[26]   Schneeweis C, Schnackenburg B, Stuber M, et al. Delayed contrast-enhanced MRI of the coronary artery wall in takayasu arteritis. *PLoS One,* 2012;7:e50655.

[27] Frias JC, Williams KJ, Fisher EA, Fayad ZA. Recombinant HDL-like nanoparticles: a specific contrast agent for MRI of atherosclerotic plaques. *J. Am. Chem. Soc.*, 2004;126:16316-7.

[28] Corti R. Noninvasive imaging of atherosclerotic vessels by MRI for clinical assessment of the effectiveness of therapy. *Pharmacol. Ther.*, 2006;110:57-70.

[29] Cyrus T, Lanza GM, Wickline SA. Molecular imaging by cardiovascular MR. *J. Cardiovasc. Magn. Reson.*, 2007;9:827-43.

[30] Spuentrup E, Katoh M, Wiethoff AJ, et al. Molecular coronary MR imaging of human thrombi using EP-2104R, a fibrin-targeted contrast agent: experimental study in a swine model. *Rofo,* 2007;179:1166-73.

[31] Spuentrup E, Botnar RM, Wiethoff AJ, et al. MR imaging of thrombi using EP-2104R, a fibrin-specific contrast agent: initial results in patients. *Eur. Radiol.,* 2008.

[32] Korosoglou G, Weiss RG, Kedziorek DA, et al. Noninvasive detection of macrophage-rich atherosclerotic plaque in hyperlipidemic rabbits using "positive contrast" magnetic resonance imaging. *J. Am. Coll. Cardiol.,* 2008;52:483-91.

[33] Temme S, Bonner F, Schrader J, Flogel U. 19F magnetic resonance imaging of endogenous macrophages in inflammation. *Wiley Interdiscip. Rev. Nanomed. Nanobiotechnol.,* 2012;4:329-43.

[34] Schachinger V, Britten MB, Zeiher AM. Prognostic impact of coronary vasodilator dysfunction on adverse long-term outcome of coronary heart disease. *Circulation,* 2000;101:1899-906.

[35] Bedaux WL, Hofman MB, de Cock CC, Stoel MG, Visser CA, van Rossum AC. Magnetic resonance imaging versus Doppler guide wire in the assessment of coronary flow reserve in patients with coronary artery disease. *Coron. Artery Dis.,* 2002;13:365-72.

[36] Hays AG, Hirsch GA, Kelle S, Gerstenblith G, Weiss RG, Stuber M. Noninvasive visualization of coronary artery endothelial function in healthy subjects and in patients with coronary artery disease. *J. Am. Coll. Cardiol.,* 2010;56:1657-65.

[37] Hays AG, Kelle S, Hirsch GA, et al. Regional coronary endothelial function is closely related to local early coronary atherosclerosis in patients with mild coronary artery disease: pilot study. *Circ. Cardiovasc. Imaging.,* 2012;5:341-8.

[38] Sathyanarayana S, Schar M, Kraitchman DL, Bottomley PA. Towards real-time intravascular endoscopic magnetic resonance imaging. *JACC Cardiovasc. Imaging.,* 2010;3:1158-65.

In: Percutaneous Coronary Intervention  ISBN: 978-1-62618-962-1
Editors: Huili Gan and Yujie Zhou  © 2013 Nova Science Publishers, Inc.

*Chapter III*

# Inner Catheter Use for Coronary Angioplasty

*Takashi Ashikaga**
Department of Cardiovascular Medicine, Tokyo Medical
and Dental University, Tokyo, Japan

## Abstract

The principle of inner catheter is to combine the advantages afforded
by the passive support of a large guide catheter with the ability to further
insert a smaller guide catheter within the target vessel, without damaging
the arterial segment proximal to the lesion. By using inner catheter, not
only stent delivery but also thrombus aspiration can be accomplished in
daily practice. Deep engagement and proper alignment of inner catheter is
necessary to deliver a stent or balloon distally and aspirate much
thrombus burden. In addition, deep engagement of a inner catheter can be
accomplished with anchor technique and/or distal balloon deflation
technique. Since inner catheter can be easily deep-engaged within and
beyond the deployed proximal stent by using distal balloon deflation
technique, proximal stent delivery followed by distal stent deployment
can be accomplished in multiple stent deployment. As with the use of
inner catheter, care withdrawing and introducing balloons and stents is

* Email: ashikaga.cvm@tmd.ac.jp. Tel: 81-3-5803-5231, Fax:81-3-5803-0133.

considered to avoid sucking air into the catheter which can be injected distally.

# Medical Use of Inner Catheter

An inner catheter has been developed for difficult stent delivery cases because it is particularly helpful if increased backup force is needed during the procedure when the wire has already been inserted with difficulty through a guide catheter of conventional length. Previous reports showed that nearly 5% of lesions could not be successfully treated with the drug-eluting stents (DES) [1]. Although many techniques of stent delivery have been developed for difficult situations [2-4], the inner catheter has remained one of the good strategies. In addition, an inner catheter has been developed for other purposes which were thrombus aspiration and the retrieval of filter wire in STEMI. Recently, both 5F and 4F inner catheter are available in daily practice. Both inner catheters have advantages and disadvantages, so it is important to know the characteristics of both inner catheters.

# The Characteristic of Inner Catheters

## The Specifications of 5F and 4F Inner Catheters

The specifications of the 5F and 4F inner catheters were shown in Table 1. Cokatte (a 4F inner catheter by Asahi Intec) cannot be used in combination with a 5F mother catheter because the outer diameter of Cokatte is 1.50mm.

**Table 1.**

| Inner catheter | | Length | Outer diameter | Inner diameter |
|---|---|---|---|---|
| 5F | Heartrail II® (Terumo) | 120 | 1.73mm | 1.50mm |
| | Dio$^{TM}$ (Goodman) | 124 | 1.73mm | 1.51mm |
| | i-works(Medikit) | 110 | 1.73mm | 1.50mm |
| 4F | Kiwami(Terumo) | 120 | 1.43mm | 1.27mm |
| | Cokatte(Asahi Intec) | 120 | 1.50mm | 1.27mm |
| | i-works (Medikit) | 120 | 1.43mm | 1.27mm |

4F i-works is available in combination with a 5F i-works because the length of a 5F i-works is 110cm. The length of 5F and 4F inner catheter is around 120cm, which is 20cm longer compared   with a conventional mother guide catheters as usual.

## Which Stents be Able to Deploy Within 5F and 4F Inner Catheters

Any bare metal stent can be deployed within a 5F inner catheter. The type of DES, which is able to deploy within a 4F inner catheter using conventional 0.014-inch guidewire is a diameter up to 3.5mm for Taxus Liberte, Resolute Integrity, Xience Prime and Promus Element and 3.0mm Nobori stent. All types of DES could be deployed by using 0.010-inch guidewire instead of 0.014-inch guidewire.

# How to Use Inner Catheter

After the failure of stent delivery using conventional technique, Y-connector was disconnected from the mother guide catheter and a small haemostatic valve was connected. Then an inner catheter is passed through the mother guide catheter along the guidewire. Y connector is re-attached to the end of an inner catheter and the interventional procedure was performed in the usual manner.

## Direct Engagement (Figure 1A)

An inner catheter is advanced into the vessel either over a coronary wire, or a wire and a balloon catheter with the balloon uninflated in the distal vessel. After the failure of stent delivery with direct engagement of an inner catheter, anchor technique and distal balloon deflation technique were employed. The most important point is not strong push of an inner catheter to prevent a guide catheter vessel injury.

## Anchor Technique (Figure1B)

At first, the balloon is placed at the distal culprit lesion. Then the balloon is inflated at 4 to 6 atm to insert an inner catheter slowly. By using the anchor technique between a balloon and an inner catheter, deep intubation of an inner catheter could be accomplished [2]. The final position of an inner catheter is placed proximal to the inflated balloon.

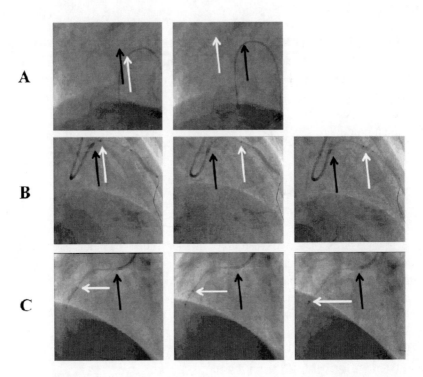

Figure 1. A: Direct engagement B: Anchor technique C:Distal balloon deflation technique. Black arrows indicate the position of mother guide catheters and whire arrows indicate the position of inner catheters.

## Distal Balloon Deflation Technique (Figure 1C)

At first, a balloon is placed at the distal culprit lesion and an inner catheter is also placed at the proximal lesion. Just after the deflation of a balloon, an inner catheter could be passed beyond the inflated balloon [5].

The final position of an inner catheter is placed distal to the inflated balloon. The distal balloon deflation technique may temporarily change orientation of the proximal section in a favorable way, which allows passage of the proximal stent and guide catheter without higher backup force. By using this technique, inner catheter can be engaged deeply within and beyond the deployed stent.

# When to Use Inner Catheter

## Procedural Characteristics

### Difficult Stent Delivery Cases

Indications for the use of an inner catheter in difficult stent delivery are severe tortuosity, severe calcification, poor backup support and trapping of the stent proximal to the target lesion (Figure2).

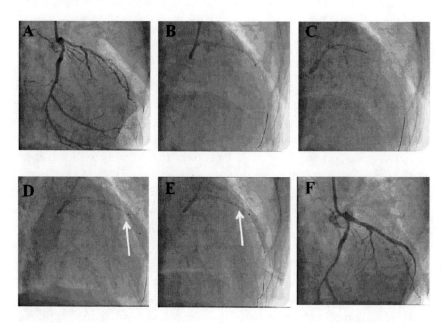

Figure 2. A: Coronary angiogram showing severe stenosis in mid LAD. B: POBA was performed at the culprit lesion. C: A 4F inner catheter could be deep engaged with anchor technique. E: DES could be delivered easily within a 4F inner catheter. F: Final angiogram. White arrows indicate the position of 4F inner catheter.

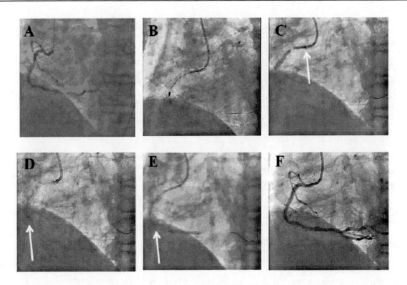

Figure 3. A: Coronary angiogram showing severe stenosis in distal RCA and severe calcification in proximal RCA. B: Rotational atherectomy (1.75mm burr) was applied at the proximal lesion. C: DES was deployed at the proximal lesion with mother-child technique. D: A 4F inner catheter was deeply engaged with distal balloon deflation technique. E: DES was deployed within a 4F inner catheter. F: Final angiogram. White arrows indicate the position of 4F inner catheter.

Prior techniques that are not effective for stent delivery are the deep engagement of mother guide catheters, the buddy wire technique and rotational atherectomy. 5F and 4F inner catheter are now available in daily practice. The principle of inner catheter is to combine the advantages afforded by the passive support of a large guide catheter with the ability to further insert a smaller guide catheter within the target vessel, without damaging the arterial segment proximal to the lesion [3, 4, 6, 7]. The soft end portion of the inner catheter can easily negotiate the tortuous coronary vessel without vessel injury. Extra deep intubation with a 5F inner catheter facilitates a stent delivery by transversing proximal points of obstruction and by increasing backup [8, 9]. Previous reports showed that increased backup force could be obtained by using 5 in 6 system compared with using 6F alone [3]. However, a 5F inner catheter often can't be advanced into an angulated calcified lesion because of a big profile. In these cases, a 4F inner catheter is a good option for the stent delivery. In addition, stent delivery for distal coronary vessel will be the target for a 4F inner catheter because a 4F inner catheter can be engaged distally compared with a 5F inner catheter. A 4F inner catheter would make the catheter more deliverable and potentially reduce the possibility for complications such as vessel injury, although at the expense of a reduced backup support and limitation of the diameter of stent that could be accommodated [10]. The proper alignment of both a 4F inner catheter and mother catheter may be important for stent delivery because limited backup force compared with a 5F inner catheter [11]. Several techniques such as anchor technique and distal balloon deflation technique should be required to advance a 4F inner catheter distally [2, 5]. In general, distal stent deployed should always be performed before proximal ones because of the risk of stent loss and/or stent dislodgement. By using the distal balloon deflation technique, an inner catheter could be easily deep-engaged within and beyond the deployed proximal stent. In this situation, a stent could be easily deployed distally within an inner catheter (Figure 3).

## *Aspiration of Thrombus*

Intracoronary thrombectomy as adjunct to stenting during direct angioplasty for STEMI was demonstrated to be effective in view of myocardial reperfusion, as assessed by myocardial blush and ST resolution [12].

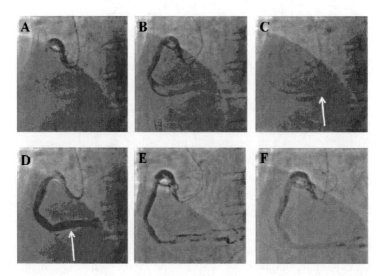

Figure 4. A: Coronary angiogram showing coronary ectasia and total occlusion in the proximal RCA. B: After thrombus aspiration catheter was applied, coronary angiogram still showed massive thrombus. C: A 5F inner catheter was deeply engaged with direct engagement. Thrombus aspiration could be performed with a 5F inner catheter directly. D: After thrombus aspiration with a 5F inner catheter. E:Final angiogrm. F: Follow up angiogram after warfarin therapy. White arrows indicate the position of 5F inner catheter.

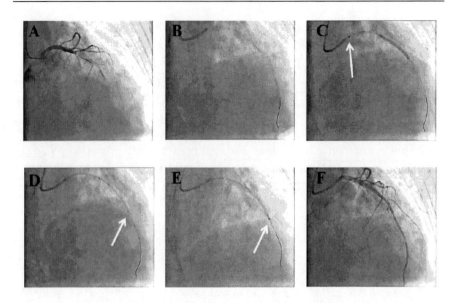

Figure 5. A: Coronary angiogram showing subtotal occlusion at the mid LAD. B:After POBA, filter wire was placed at the distal LAD. C: BMS was deployed at the culprit lesion with 4 in 6 system. D:After BMS implantation, a 4F inner catheter was deeply engaged beyond the deployed stent. E: Retrieval of filter wire and thrombus aspiration were accomplished with a 4F inner catheter. Final angiogram. White arrows indicate the position of 4F inner catheter.

In addition, management using a combined thrombus aspiration catheter and filter wire approach was shown to result in an excellent clinical outcome for cases with thrombotic burden [13]. If the much thrombus has been stayed within the coronary artery, it is effective to aspirate directly from the inner catheter because inner catheter, which has a big profile compared to the aspiration catheter, has to be deep engaged (Figure 4).

Retrieval of filter wire also could be performed by using the distal balloon deflation technique. Briefly, a stent was deployed with the mother-child technique. When the stent was deployed, inner catheter should be placed proximal to the stent. Just after the deflation of the stent balloon, the inner catheter could be deeply engaged within and beyond the deployed stent by using distal balloon deflation technique. Both stent delivery and thrombus aspiration can be accomplished simultaneously. In addition, retrieval of filter wire also could be performed easily without the risk of entrapment by the deployed stent because inner catheter was placed beyond the deployed stent [11] (Figure5).

### Retrieval of Entrapped or Retained Equipments

If an equipment is retained or entrapped within a coronary artery, this can lead to myocardial ischemia, infarction, and lethal arrhythmias [14, 15]. Various percutaneous retrieval methods have already been described in the literature: loop snare, dormia basket, double or triple guidewire technique, hocked guidewire, forgaty balloon, bronchoscopic forceps, and cardiac biotome [16-20]. Although a variety of techniques have been introduced in these situations, most of them have been time and cost consuming methods. In addition, none of these techniques have emerged as the best retrieval modality. By using another guidewire, it is sometimes possible to wrap or twist two or three guidewires to entire the junk and then withdraw it into a guide catheter. In addition, recrossing another guidewire just beside the entrapped burr and making a crack between the burr and vessel wall by inflating a balloon catheter might be a more promising strategy in entrapped rotational atherectomy burr [21, 22].

Arguably, different techniques may be better suited for a particular mechanism of entrapment such as rotablator entrapment.

# Adverse Effects and Complication of Inner Catheter

The most important adverse effect is the pressure damping occurring when an inner catheter is advanced distally.

Finally limited lumen size of 5F inner catheter (0.059 inch) limits the stent size. In addition, as with the use of the 4F inner catheter, care withdrawing and introducing balloons and stents is considered to avoid sucking air into the catheter which can be injected distally. In addition, limited lumen size of 4F inner catheter (0.050 inch) limits the stent size and type compared with 5F inner catheters.

## Technical Issue

### How to Withdraw an Inner Catheter

Using an extension guidewire, inner catheters are withdrawn from the coronary system.

The Nanto method is also effective in removing inner catheters from the coronary system. Briefly, the Nanto method is used after the entrance of microcatheter, and a connection between inner catheters and microcatheters should be required.

# References

[1]   Morice MC, Colombo A, Meier B. Serruys P, Tamburino C, Guagliumi G, Sousa E, Stol HP. Sirolimus- vs Paclitaxel- eluting stents in de novo coronary artery lesions. *JAMA,* 2006;295:895-904.
[2]   Fujita S, Tamai H, Kyo E, Kosuga K, Hata T, Okada M, Nakamura T, Tsuji T, Takeda S, Bin HF, Masunaga N, Motohara S, Uehata H. New technique for superior guiding catheter support during advancement of a balloon in coronary angioplasty: the anchor technique. *Catheter Cardiovasc. Interv.,* 2003;59:482-488.
[3]   Takahashi S, Saito S, Tanaka S, Miyashita Y, Shiono T, Arai F, Domae H, Satake S, Ito T. New method to increase a backup support of a 6 french guiding catheter. *Catheter Cardiovasc. Interv.,* 2004;63:452-456.
[4]   Ashikaga T, Nishizaki M, Yamawake N. Difficult stent delivery: Use of an aspiration catheter as a " sheath". *Catheter Cardiovasc. Interv.,* 2008;71:909-912.
[5]   Ashikaga T, Sakurai K, Satoh Y. Distal balloon deflation technique: a new method to facilitate entry of balloon catheter, stent and guiding catheter to distal lesion. *Catheter Cardiovasc. Interv.,* 2010;75:356-361.
[6]   Garcia-Garcia HM, Kukreja N, Daemon J, Shuzou T, Van Mieghem C, Gonzalo N, van Weenen S, van der Ent M, Sianos G, de Feyter P, Serruys PW. Contemporary treatment of patients with chronic total occlusion: critical appraisal of different state of the art techniques and devices. *Eurointervention,* 2007;3:E1-9.
[7]   Shaukat A, Al-Bustami M, Ong PJ. Chronic total occlusion- use of a 5 french guiding catheter in a 6 french guiding catheter. *J. Invasive Cardiol.,* 2008;20:317-318.
[8]   Mamas MA, Fath-Ordoubadi F, Fraser D. Successful use of the Heartrail II catheter as a stent delivery catheter following failure of conventional technique. *Catheter Cardiovasc. Interv.,* 2008;71:358-363.
[9]   Mamas MA, Eichhofer J, Hendry C, El-Omar M, Clarke B, Neyses l, Fath-Ordoubadi F, Frase D. Use of the Heartrail II catheter as a distal stent delivery device; an extended case series. *Eurointervention,* 2009;5:265-271.

[10] Ashikaga T, Sakurai K, Satoh Y. Tools and techniques; Stent delivery in distal lesions. *Eurointervention,* 2010;6:660-661.

[11] Ashikaga T, Sakurai K, Satoh Y. A novel mother and child technique with a 4F inner catheter based on proper alignment of both catheters. *Catheter Cardiovasc. Interv.,* 2012;79:1004-1008.

[12] Napodano M, Pasquetto G, Saccà S, Cernetti C, Scarabeo V, Pascotto P, Reimers B. Intracoronary thrombectomy improves myocardial reperfusion in patients undergoing direct angioplasty for acute myocardial infarction. *J. Am. Coll. Cardiol.,* 2003;42:1395-1402.

[13] Moharram MA, Brieger D, Lowe HC. Feasibility of using the export catheter monorailed over filterwire for native coronary intervention in the presence of thrombus. *Int. J. Cardiol.,* 2009;137:e49-e50.

[14] Kuruma A, Saitoh H, Ino T, Atarashi H, Katoh T, Hayakawa H, Ikeshita M, Tanaka S. Case of cardiac foreign bodies associated with four types of tachycardias. *Pacing. Clin. Electrophysiol.,* 1992;15:1215-1224.

[15] Breisblatt WM. Inflated balloon entrapped in a calcified coronary stenosis. *Catheter Cardiovasc. Diagn.,* 1993;29:224-228.

[16] Hartzler GO, Rutherford BD, McConathay DR. Retained percutaneous trasluminal coronary angioplasty equipment components and their management. *Am. J. Cardiol.,* 1987;60:1260-1264.

[17] Gurley JC, Booth DC, Hixson C, Smith MD. Removal of retained intracoronary percutaneous coronary angioplasty equipment by a percutaneous twin guidewire method. *Catheter Cardiovasc. Diagn.,* 1990;19:251-256.

[18] Collins N, Horlick E, Dzavik V. Triple wire technique for removal of fractured angioplasty guidewire. *J. Invasive Cardiol.,* 2007;19:E230-234.

[19] Hung CL, Tsai CT, Hou CJY. Percutaneous transcatheter retrieval of retained balloon catheter in distal tortuous coronary artery: a modified double-herix approach. *Catheter Cardiovasc. Interv.,* 2004;62:471-475.

[20] Patel T, Shah S, Pandya R, Sanghvi K, Fonseca K. Broken guidewire fragment: a simplified retrieval technique. *Catheter Cardiovasc. Interv.,* 2000;51:483-486.

[21] Grise MA, Yeager MJ, Teirstein PS. A case of an entrapped rotational atheterctomy burr. *Catheter Cardiovasc. Interv.,* 2002;57:31-33.

[22] Hyogo M, Inoue N, Nakamura R, Tokura T, Matsuo A, Inoue K, Tanaka K, Fujita H. Usefulness of conquest guidewire for retrieval of an entrapped rotablator burr. *Catheter Cardiovasc. Interv.,* 2004;63:469-472.

In: Percutaneous Coronary Intervention          ISBN: 978-1-62618-962-1
Editors: Huili Gan and Yujie Zhou          © 2013 Nova Science Publishers, Inc.

*Chapter IV*

# Nucleic Acid Drugs to Prevent Restenosis after Coronary Intervention: From Bench to Bedside

*Jun-ichi Suzuki[1]\*, Ryuichi Morishita[2],*
*Yasunobu Hirata[1] and Mitsuaki Isobe[3]*
[1]Department of Advanced Clinical Science and Therapeutics,
University of Tokyo, Tokyo, Japan
[2]Department of Clinical Gene Therapy, Osaka University, Osaka, Japan
[3]Department of Cardiovascular Medicine,
Tokyo Medical and Dental University, Tokyo, Japan

## Abstract

Nuclear factor-kappa B (NF-κB) plays a pivotal role in restenosis after percutaneous coronary intervention (PCI). To evaluate the effectiveness of an NF-κB decoy oligodeoxynucleotide (ODN) for

\* Correspondence to Jun-ichi Suzuki, Department of Advanced Clinical Science and Therapeutics, Graduate School of Medicine, University of Tokyo, 7-3-1 Hongo, Bunkyo, Tokyo 113-8655, Japan; phone 81-3-5800-9116, fax 81-3-5800-9182, e-mail junichisuzuki-circ@umin.ac.jp.

preventing restenosis, we performed experimental studies and clinical trials. Firstly, we performed *in vivo* NF-κB decoy ODN transfection in murine injured arteries. Murine femoral arteries were injured using flexible wires. Pathologically, the NF-κB decoy ODN transfection group showed smaller neointima per media area ratios than those in the control groups. Immunohistochemistry revealed that enhanced expression of inflammatory factors was observed in non-treated injured arteries, while the NF-κB decoy ODN suppressed the expression. Based on these experimental results, we initiated an open label phase I/IIa clinical trial to evaluate the safety and effectiveness of NF-κB decoy ODN. Seventeen patients, who were suffering from angina, were treated with NF-κB decoy ODN after PCI using bare metal stents. Three days after PCI, serum MCP-1 levels were significantly suppressed in NF-κB decoy ODN treated patients compared to the non-treated patients. Six months after PCI and decoy ODN transfection, significant restenosis was found in only 1 of the 17 patients. In-stent thrombosis was not found and no significant systemic adverse effect occurred in any of the patients in the six-months observation period. One of the 17 cases has been regularly examined for eight years after ODN transfection. We revealed that decoy ODN treatment suppressed neointimal formation in comparison to the stent lesion without ODN transfection in the same artery. Thus, we showed the safety and long-term usefulness of NF-κB decoy ODN transfer after PCI.

# Introduction

The major disadvantage of percutaneous coronary intervention (PCI) in the treatment of patients with atherosclerotic coronary disease is the occurrence of restenosis and thrombus formation [1].

Although drug eluting stents (DES) have been broadly used to prevent restenosis [2], long-term usage of anti-platelet drugs is needed to prevent thrombus formation [3, 4]. Experimental studies and clinical histology have demonstrated that thrombus formation is caused by delayed endothelialization of the coronary arteries. This is because conservative DES distributes immunosuppressive or anticartinogenic drugs to the PCI cites [5]. Therefore, prevention of restenosis without delayed endothelialization is needed for clinical PCI.

Neointimal formation and endothelialization is developed by accumulation of leukocyte and hematopoietic stem cells in the arterial wall [6]. Nuclear factor-kappa B (NF-κB) is critical in the coordinated gene transactivation of cytokines and adhesion molecules. The synthetic double-stranded DNA with high affinity for NF-κB, which is known as a 'decoy oligodeoxynucleotides (ODN)', has specific effects on the suppression of inflammatory factors. The decoy ODN strategy significantly effects the treatment of acute myocardial infarction [7] and cardiac rejection [8]. We also demonstrated that NF-κB decoy ODN inhibited neointimal formation after arterial balloon injury [9, 10]. Because NF-κB decoy ODN provide a new therapeutic strategy to treat cardiovascular disease [11], we initiated open label phase I/IIa clinical trial to evaluate the safety and efficacy of NF-κB decoy ODN. In this review article, we demonstrate the effectiveness of an NF-κB decoy ODN for preventing restenosis using experimental studies and clinical trials.

# Experimental Studies

We made a murine arterial injury model as described previously [12]. Endothelial denudation injury of the artery was performed by use of wire withdrawal injury. Three passes were made along the artery. To confirm the in vivo efficacy of NF-κB decoy ODN on the prevention of neointimal formation, we used the murine arterial injury model and the ultrasound-microbubble method.

Immediately after arterial injury, 90 µl of the NF-κB decoy ODN (20 µg) plus microbubble (10 µl) mixture was suspended in echo gel (300 µl) and applied to the perivascular surface of the arteries. The ultrasound was irradiated for 30 seconds (1 MHz, 1.0 W/cm2, duty 20 %) [13]. The arteries were harvested on day 14 and then stained with hematoxylin and eosin (HE) and Elastica van Gieson (EvG). The severity of intimal thickening was quantitatively assessed in each artery as described earlier [14]. We found that the NF-κB decoy ODN with microbubble plus ultrasound group showed suppressed neointimal formation compared to the control groups. To clarify the mechanism, we performed immunohistochemistry. Expression of MOMA-2, ICAM-1 and PCNA was enhanced in the thickened intima of the injured arteries in the control groups. In contrast, the expression was reduced in the arteries from mice which received the NF-κB decoy ODN with microbubble plus ultrasound [14].

# A Clinical Trial

Patients with stable angina pectoris or silent ischemia with a single de novo organic stenosis lesion in a native coronary artery were enrolled. Bare metal stents were implanted into the coronary stenotic sites. NF-κB decoy ODN (1, 2 or 4 mg per body) was trasnfected using the Remedy catheter (Boston Scientific); the solution (0.5 mL) was administered manually with 100kPa. Its delivery took 50 seconds for the delivery. A coronary angiogram with quantitative coronary angiography (QCA) and intravenous ultrasound (IVUS) were performed before and immediately after the stent implantation, and 6 months after the treatment. Peripheral blood was examined from patients on days 0, 1, 3, and 7 after the treatment to determine the serum concentration of monocyte chemoattractant protein (MCP)-1. All cases successfully received stent implantation and decoy ODN transfection without initial complications. The serum levels of MCP-1 were less in the decoy ODN treated group compared to the non-decoy ODN treated group. Seventeen cases received all examinations during this 6 months period. As only 1 of the 17 patients showed significant stenosis (more than 75%), the average stenosis rate was less than 40%. In-stent thrombosis and major adverse effect were not found during this observation period [15, 16].

We followed some of the cases in our outpatient clinics. The first case was followed for more than 8 years and there was no ischemic event and adverse effects. A 53-year-old man presented at our hospital suffering from chest pain after exertion. Although he had received PCI with many metallic stents several times; he continued to experience restenosis. Conventional coronary angiography revealed high-grade stenosis in the proximal (#1) and middle (#2) portions of the right coronary artery. He received a PCI with two metallic stent implantations at both stenotic sites. We delivered the NF-κB decoy ODN at the distal site (#2) and no decoy at the proximal site (#1). Six months after PCI and NF-κB decoy delivery, QCA and IVUS were performed to evaluate the coronary artery for restenosis at the stent implantation sites. IVUS revealed that the NF-κB decoy ODN treatment suppressed the development of neointimal formation (#2) compared to the non-decoy ODN transfection site (#1). On year 4 and 8 after the PCI and NF-κB decoy ODN delivery, CT scans were performed to evaluate the coronary artery for restenosis at the stent implantation sites. The scan revealed that NF-κB decoy ODN treatment suppressed the development of neointimal formation (#2) compared to the non-decoy ODN transfection site (#1). We assessed the degree of stenosis and compared the values between year 4 and 8 after stent implantation. The analysis showed that there was a difference between non-decoy ODN lesion (57.9%) and NF-κB decoy ODN lesion (28.8%) on year 8. It is noteworthy that there was no progression of restenosis at the NF-κB decoy ODN lesion site. The degrees of restenosis in the NF-κB decoy ODN area were comparable between year 4 and year 8. Systemic adverse effects and late thrombosis formation were not observed during this period [17, 18].

# Discussion

This is an article to report the successful transfection of NF-κB decoy ODN at the site of vascular intervention. These experimental and clinical findings suggest safe and favorable effects of NF-κB decoy ODN on the prevention of restenosis after PCI. Although DES has been used to prevent restenosis after PCI, in-stent thrombosis has yet to be resolved. The thrombosis is caused by delayed re-endothelialization of the inner layer of the stent-implanted arteries. This is because DES elutes strong immunosuppressants and anti-cancer drugs into the injured artery. These drugs suppress the proliferation of arterial endothelial and smooth muscle cells [19-21]. Thus, a new strategy to prevent both restenosis and thrombus formation is needed in the near future.

Inflammation is an essential pathological feature of neointimal formation, NF-κB plays an important role in this process [22]. Thus, NF-κB regulation has the potential to suppress the progression of inflammation. Decoy ODN transfection is a significant methodology for suppressing gene activation. NF-κB decoy ODN is double stranded DNA with specific affinity to the cis-element of NF-κB, thereby leading to the suppression of many inflammatory factors, including adhesion molecules and cytokines [23]. Therefore, NF-κB decoy ODN transfection at the stent site suppressed smooth muscle cell proliferation, which resulted in less neointimal formation. NF-κB decoy ODN might serve the re-endothelialization to a satisfactory degree, because NF-κB decoy ODN inhibited the apoptosis of endothelial cells in response to hypoxia [24]. Indeed, the transfection of NF-κB decoy ODN into a vein graft demonstrated the significant improvement of endothelial dysfunction as compared to control [25]. Thus, NF-κB decoy ODN strategy may avoid the long-term anti-platelet therapy that prevents late thrombosis.

We showed that NF-κB decoy ODN transfection suppressed serum MCP-1 levels compared to those in the control group. As previously reported, MCP-1 production at stent-implanted coronary arterial sites is associated with an increased risk for restenosis [26].

Thus, our findings suggest that this novel treatment may benefit the prevention of restenosis after PCI. These data suggest that this strategy is practical and promising for the prevention of in-stent restenosis and thrombus formation in humans.

# References

[1]    Leimgruber PP, Roubin GS, Hollman J, et al. Restenosis after successful coronary angioplasty in patients with single-vessel disease. Circulation 1986; 73: 710-717.

[2]    Haude M, Konorza TF, Kalnins U, et al. Heparin-coated stent placement for the treatment of stenoses in small coronary arteries of symptomatic patients. Circulation 2003; 107: 1265-1270.

[3]    Holmes DR Jr. In-stent restenosis. Rev Cardiovasc Med 2001; 2: 115-119.

[4]    Danzi GB, Sesana M, Capuano C, Predolini S, Baglini R. Restenosis after NIR stent implantation. Minerva Cardioangiol 2002; 50: 455-462.

[5]    Wilensky RL, March KL, Gradus-Pizlo I, Sandusky G, Fineberg N, Hathaway DR. Vascular injury, repair, and restenosis after percutaneous transluminal angioplasty in the atherosclerotic rabbit. Circulation 1995; 92: 2995-3005.

[6]    Sata M, Saiura A, Kunisato A, et al. Hematopoietic stem cells differentiate into vascular cells that participate in the pathogenesis of atherosclerosis. Nat Med 2002; 8: 403-409.

[7]    Morishita R, Sugimoto T, Aoki M, et al. In vivo transfection of cis element "decoy" against nuclear factor-kappaB binding site prevents myocardial infarction. Nat Med 1997; 3: 894-899.

[8]    Suzuki J, Morishita R, Amano J, Kaneda Y, Isobe M. Decoy against nuclear factor-kappa B attenuates myocardial cell infiltration and arterial neointimal formation in murine cardiac allografts. Gene Ther 2000; 7: 1847-1852.

[9]    Yoshimura S, Morishita R, Hayashi K, et al. Inhibition of intimal hyperplasia after balloon injury in rat carotid artery model using cis-

element 'decoy' of nuclear factor-kappaB binding site as a novel molecular strategy. Gene Ther 2001; 8: 1635-1642.

[10] Yamasaki K, Asai T, Shimizu M, et al. Inhibition of NF-κB activation using cis-element "decoy" of NF-κB binding site reduces neointimal formation in porcine balloon-injured coronary artery model. Gene Ther 2003; 10: 356-364.

[11] Morishita R. Recent progress in gene therapy for cardiovascular disease. Circ J 2002; 66: 1077-1086.

[12] Lindner V, Fingerle J, Reidy MA. Mouse model of arterial injury. Circ Res 1993; 73: 792-796.

[13] Nakashima H, Aoki M, Miyake T, Kawasaki T, Iwai M, Jo N, Oishi M, Kataoka K, Ohgi S, Ogihara T, Kaneda Y, Morishita R. Inhibition of experimental abdominal aortic aneurysm in the rat by use of decoy oligodeoxynucleotides suppressing activity of nuclear factor kappaB and ets transcription factors. Circulation 2004; 109: 132-8.

[14] Inagaki H, Suzuki J, Ogawa M, Taniyama Y, Morishita R, Isobe M. Ultrasound-microbubble mediated NF-kB decoy transfection attenuates neointimal formation after arterial injury in mice. J Vasc Res 2006; 43: 12-18.

[15] Suzuki J, Ito H, Gotoh R, Morishita R, Egashira K, Isobe M. Initial clinical cases using an NF-kB decoy at the site of the coronary stenting for prevention of restenosis. Circ J 2004; 68: 270-1.

[16] Egashira K, Suzuki J, Ito H, Aoki M, Isobe M, Morishita R, for INDOR Study Group. Long-term follow up of initial clinical cases with NF-kB decoy oligodeoxynucleotide transfection at the site of the coronary stenting. J Gene Med 2008; 10: 805-809.

[17] Suzuki J, Tezuka D, Morishita R, Isobe M. An initial case of suppressed restenosis with NF-kB decoy transfection after PCI. J Gene Med 2009; 11: 89-91.

[18] Suzuki J, Tezuka D, Morishita R, Isobe M. Eight-year follow-up of an initial case with NF-kB decoy oligodeoxynucleotide transfection after coronary stent implantation. Immun Endoc Metab Agents in Med Chem 2012; 12: 40-2.

[19] Luscher TF, Steffel J, Eberli FR, et al. Drug-eluting stent and coronary thrombosis: biological mechanisms and clinical implications. Circulation 2007; 115: 1051-1058.

[20] Pasceri V, Patti G, Speciale G, Pristipino C, Richichi G, Di Sciascio G. Meta-analysis of clinical trials on use of drug-eluting stents for treatment of acute myocardial infarction. Am Heart J 2007; 153: 749-754.

[21] Leon MB. Late thrombosis a concern with drug-eluting stents. J Interv Cardiol 2007; 20: 26-29.

[22] Squadrito F, Deodato B, Bova A, et al. Crucial role of nuclear factor-kappaB in neointimal hyperplasia of the mouse carotid artery after interruption of blood flow. Atherosclerosis 2003; 166: 233-242.

[23] Yokoseki O, Suzuki J, Kitabayashi H, et al. cis element decoy against neculear factor-kB attenuates development of experimental autoimmune myocarditis in rats. Circ Res 2001; 89: 899-906.

[24] Matsushita H, Morishita R, Nata T, et al. Hypoxia-induced endothelial apoptosis through nuclear factor-kappaB (NF-kappaB)-mediated bcl-2 suppression: in vivo evidence of the importance of NF-kappaB in endothelial cell regulation. Circ Res 2000; 86: 974-981.

[25] Miyake T, Aoki M, Shiraya S, et al. Inhibitory effects of NF-κB decoy oligodeoxynucleotides on neointimal hyperplasia in a rabbit vein graft model. J Mol Cell Cardiol 2006; 41: 431-440.

[26] Oshima S, Ogawa H, Hokimoto S, et al. Plasma monocyte chemoattractant protein-1 antigen levels and the risk of restenosis after coronary stent implantation. Jpn Circ J 2001; 65: 261-264.

In: Percutaneous Coronary Intervention          ISBN: 978-1-62618-962-1
Editors: Huili Gan and Yujie Zhou          © 2013 Nova Science Publishers, Inc.

*Chapter V*

# Pharmacological Agents during Percutaneous Coronary Intervention

*David C. Yang, Rajesh V. Swaminathan,*
*Luke K. Kim and Dmitriy N. Feldman* *
Weill Cornell Medical College, New York Presbyterian Hospital,
New York, New York, US

## Abstract

The benefits of percutaneous coronary intervention (PCI) can be offset by peri-procedural complications such as acute vessel closure and stent thrombosis (ST) in the absence of adequate antiplatelet and anticoagulation therapy.

Additionally, conditions occurring after 30 days post-PCI, such as in-stent restenosis or late ST can occur. Excess antithrombotic therapy on the other hand carries a risk of major gastrointestinal or intracranial bleeding as well as vascular access site bleeding complications. In this

* Address for correspondence and reprints: Dmitriy N. Feldman, MD, Assistant Professor of Medicine, Weill Cornell Medical College, New York Presbyterian Hospital, Department of Medicine, Greenberg Division of Cardiology, 520 East 70th Street, Starr-434 Pavilion, New York, NY 10021, Phone: (212) 746-4644; Fax: (212) 746-8295, Email: dnf9001@med.cornell.edu.

chapter, evidence related to the various pharmacological agents available to clinicians during and after PCI will be explored.

# Introduction

The use of percutaneous coronary intervention (PCI) in the modern era has greatly improved patient outcomes in the face of acute myocardial infarction (MI) as well as in disabling cardiac angina, however, its benefits can be limited by peri-procedural complications such as catheter and wire associated thrombus formation, acute vessel closure and stent thrombosis (ST). Coronary stents are generally made of stainless steel or cobalt chromium alloys rendering them thrombogenic until they are completely covered by endothelial tissue.

**Table 1. ARC summary of consensus definitions for stent thrombosis**

| Definite stent thrombosis |
| --- |
| Angiographic confirmation<br>Presence of thrombus originating in the stent or in the segment 5 mm proximal or distal to the stent<br>that is associated with at least 1 of the following criteria within 48 hours of angiography:<br>Acute onset of ischemic symptoms at rest<br>Acute ischemic changes on ECG<br>Typical rise and fall of cardiac biomarkers<br>Pathologic confirmation<br>Thrombus seen within the stent at autopsy or from tissue retrieved after thrombectomy. |
| Probable stent thrombosis |
| Any unexplained death within the first 30 days following intracoronary stenting.<br>Any MI with evidence of acute ischemia in the territory of the implanted stent without angiographic<br>confirmation of stent thrombosis and without any other obvious cause, irrespective of time from index<br>stent placement. |
| Possible stent thrombosis |
| Any unexplained death occurring more than 30 days after intracoronary stenting. |

Data from: Cutlip DE, Windecker S, Mehran R, et al. on behalf of the Academic Research Consortium. Clinical end points in coronary stent trials: a case for standardized definitions. Circulation 2007; 115:2344.

**Table 2. Factors associated with increased risk of stent thrombosis**

| |
|---|
| Absence or premature discontinuation of dual anti-platelet therapy |
| High on-treatment platelet reactivity (with clopidogrel) |
| Genetic polymorphisms in hepatic enzymes involved in clopidogrel metabolism |
| Stent under-expansion |
| Greater stent length |
| Small vessel diameter |
| Inflow or outflow obstruction (>50% intracoronary stenosis) |
| Post-procedure TIMI flow grade < 3 |
| Bifurcation lesions |
| Emergent PCI or ACS |
| Residual thrombus or stent edge dissection |
| Subtherapeutic peri-procedural anticoagulation |
| Severe left ventricular dysfunction |
| History of brachytherapy |
| Cocaine use |
| Malignancy |

Adapted from: David C. Yang and Dmitriy N. Feldman (2012). Pharmacotherapy During Percutaneous Coronary Interventions, Coronary Interventions, Neville Kukreja (Ed.), ISBN: 978-953-51-0498-8, InTech, Available from: http://www.intechopen.com/books/coronary-interventions/pharmacotherapy-during-percutaneous-coronary-interventions.

The timing of complete endothelialization is variable and depends on whether the implanted stent is bare metal (BMS) or drug-eluting (DES), as well as which type of anti-proliferative drug the stent is coated with. Excess antithrombotic therapy carries a risk of major gastrointestinal or intracranial bleeding as well as bleeding complications at the vascular access site. ST is a relatively infrequent event after PCI though it remains one of the most feared complications as patients usually present with death or ST-elevation myocardial infarction (STEMI). Standardized definitions for ST exist and these include definite ST, probable ST, and possible ST (Table 1). ST can also be described based on its timing relative to stent placement. The incidence of ST is highest within the first 30 days after PCI (early ST: acute [within 24 hours] and subacute [>24 hours and <30 days]), however the risk persists up to one year (late ST) and beyond (very late ST) [1]. In one large registry study,

ST was identified in 1.8% of over 400,000 patients presenting with acute coronary syndrome (ACS) [2]. Of these, 19.6% were early ST, 19.4% were late ST, and 61.0% were very late ST. Patients with early ST had higher in-hospital mortality rates (7.9%) compared to late (3.8%) and very late ST (3.6%, p<0.001). Many factors can increase the risk of ST including clinical co-morbidities and technical issues related to stent deployment (Table 2). Diabetes, renal failure, and congestive heart failure can all increase the risk of ST by up to three-fold. Longer stent length, overlapping stents, bifurcation stenting, and malapposed stents also incur a greater risk of ST [3]. The incidence of early and late ST between BMS and DES is fairly equivalent, though there appears to be a trend toward increased very late ST with the first-generation DES, thought to be related to delayed neointimal coverage as well as ongoing vessel inflammation [4–7].

The greatest risk factor for ST, however, remains premature discontinuation of antiplatelet medications demonstrating the importance of platelet aggregation in the pathophysiology of ST and the role of antiplatelet pharmacotherapy in ST prevention. Current ACC/AHA guidelines make a number of recommendations regarding the concurrent use of antiplatelet, antithrombotic, and thrombolytic pharmacotherapy during PCI to prevent such complications. The goal of this chapter will be to describe different therapeutic agents available to clinicians during and after PCI and to summarize the most current guidelines regarding their use.

# Anti-Platelet Agents

## Aspirin

Aspirin irreversibly inactivates cyclooxygenase-1, inhibiting prostaglandin and thromboxane synthesis which in turn diminishes platelet aggregation. The effects of aspirin therapy on reducing morbidity and mortality in primary ACS have been well described dating back to the pre-PCI era [8–12]. Recommendations for its use in PCI with stenting are derived from several early clinical trials in which treatment with high dose aspirin (650 mg to 990 mg/day) along with dipyridamole or ticlopidine in percutaneous transluminal coronary angioplasty (PTCA) was compared to placebo. Patients who were treated with aspirin-based regimens uniformly had better outcomes with significant reductions in peri-procedural complications including abrupt vessel closure, dissection or MI [13]. Pretreatment with aspirin monotherapy was tested against aspirin plus dipyridamole and shown to have an independent beneficial effect [14]. Subsequent studies comparing high-dose versus low-dose aspirin (1500 mg vs. 80 mg/day) prior to PTCA showed no difference in the incidence of MI or in the rate of major complications and restenosis [15]. The most current ACC/AHA guidelines recommend that aspirin be administered as soon as possible for ACS or prior to PCI and is to be continued indefinitely in patients who tolerate it [16].

## Ticlopidine

Ticlopidine, an irreversible inhibitor of the platelet adenosine diphosphate (ADP) receptor $P2Y_{12}$, is a first-generation thienopyridine that reduces platelet activation and aggregation. The STAIG trial, one of the first to evaluate the role of thienopyridines in ACS, randomized 652 patients with unstable angina (UA) to conventional medical therapy alone versus ticlopidine in addition to conventional treatment [17]. Ticlopidine use was associated with a reduction in vascular mortality by 46.8% (4.8% vs. 8.9%) and MI by 53.2% (5.1% vs. 10.9%). Further randomized trials such as STARS, MATTIS, ISAR, and FANTASTIC compared dual antiplatelet therapy (DAPT) with ticlopidine and aspirin to conventional anticoagulant therapy with heparin or warfarin in PCI with BMS and demonstrated a clear reduction in ST, death, MI, or emergent coronary artery bypass graft (CABG) surgery [18–21]. Ticlopidine, however, has been associated with significant side effects including thrombocytopenia, neutropenia and thrombotic thrombocytopenic purpura-hemolytic uremic syndrome. Thus, its use is rare now and it is crucial that careful monitoring of blood counts be performed regularly after initiation of therapy [22, 23].

## Clopidogrel

Due to the unfavorable side effect profile of ticlopidine, interest developed in clopidogrel as a potential thienopyridine alternative. Clopidogrel, a second-generation thienopyridine, is a prodrug that requires bioactivation by the cytochrome P450 (CYP) system therefore its clinical effectiveness is altered by genetic polymorphisms and other medications that also utilize the CYP system. The efficacy of clopidogrel in the treatment of coronary artery disease (CAD) was demonstrated in the CAPRIE trial in which clopidogrel use significantly reduced the combined endpoint of ischemic stroke, MI and vascular death in patients with atherosclerotic disease [24]. Clopidogrel's overall safety benefit as compared to ticlopidine was convincingly shown in the CLASSICS trial, with a subsequent meta-analysis finding that clopidogrel use was at least as efficacious as ticlopidine with fewer major adverse cardiac events (MACE) and a lower incidence of mortality while having fewer side effects and being more tolerable for patients [25, 26]. Based on these findings, clopidogrel replaced ticlopidine as the thienopyridine of choice in combination with aspirin as standard therapy after PCI. Several landmark trials then fully expanded the application of clopidogrel therapy to ACS and PCI. The CURE trial studied 12,562 patients with non-ST-elevation ACS (NSTE-ACS) and found a 20% reduction in the primary combined endpoint of cardiovascular death, MI, or stroke (9.3% vs. 11.4%) when treated with combined aspirin and clopidogrel as compared to aspirin alone [27]. When the subset of patients undergoing PCI was analyzed separately in the PCI-CURE substudy, pretreatment with clopidogrel plus aspirin prior to PCI led to both immediate and long-term benefits in reducing ischemic vascular events and death [28, 29]. The CREDO trial later confirmed the benefit of upstream clopidogrel therapy in 2,116 patients who were randomized to receive either clopidogrel at a 300 mg loading dose or placebo 3 to 24 hours before elective PCI, followed by 75 mg daily for 28 days in both groups and then either clopidogrel or placebo out to one year according to the original randomization [30]. At one year, investigators found a 26.9% relative risk reduction in the combined end point of death, MI, or stroke (8.5% vs. 11.5%, 95% CI 3.9-44.4) with clopidogrel therapy, showing that long-term treatment with clopidogrel was beneficial. Two additional large randomized trials, CLARITY-TIMI 28 and COMMIT/CCS-2, then demonstrated that clopidogrel therapy when added to aspirin also improved outcomes in patients with STEMI being treated with fibrinolytics and heparin [31, 32].

With the role of clopidogrel now clearly defined in all forms of ACS as well as PCI, the timing and dose of optimal clopidogrel pretreatment for PCI was evaluated. In a prespecified subgroup analysis, the PCI-CLARITY trial found that early treatment with clopidogrel 300 mg led to significantly better outcomes in all time groups ranging from within 6 hours before PCI to as far as 96 hours ahead of PCI [33]. A substudy from CREDO, however, found that the benefit was only seen if clopidogrel 300 mg was given 10-12 hours before PCI and did not become significant unless given >15 hours prior to PCI, with a maximum effect seen at 24 hours [34]. Since pretreatment with clopidogrel for >15 hours prior to PCI is often impractical in situations of ACS where an early invasive strategy is planned or in ad hoc decisions to stent at the time of diagnostic angiography, higher loading doses of clopidogrel were studied and found to be beneficial by increasing the level of platelet inhibition while reaching maximum antiplatelet effects in a shorter amount of time. In an unselected cohort of over 1,000 patients who were given a 600 mg dose of clopidogrel, in vitro studies found that maximum platelet inhibition was seen by two hours with additional studies showing that 600 mg of clopidogrel achieved higher levels of peak platelet inhibition compared to the conventional 300 mg dose [35, 36]. Subsequent studies sought to evaluate whether these pharmacodynamic differences could translate into improved patient outcomes. The ARMYDA-2 trial randomized 255 patients with stable angina or NSTE-ACS to either 600 mg or 300 mg of clopidogrel given four to eight hours prior to PCI [37]. By 30 days, the composite endpoint of death, MI, or target vessel revascularization (TVR) occurred significantly less in patients treated with 600 mg versus 300 mg (4% vs. 12%), a difference that was entirely driven by rates of peri-procedural MI. No differences were reported in the rates of major bleeding between the two groups. The benefit of a clopidogrel 600 mg loading dose was seen again in a subgroup analysis from the HORIZONS-AMI landmark trial in which 3,602 patients with STEMI undergoing primary PCI were randomized to either bivalirudin or unfractionated heparin (UFH) plus a glycoprotein (GP) IIb/IIIa inhibitor [38]. Clopidogrel loading doses of either 300 mg (1,153 patients) or 600 mg (2,158 patients) were chosen at the clinician's discretion and after multivariable analysis, the 600 mg dose was found to be an independent predictor of lower rates of 30-day major adverse cardiac events (MACE) without higher bleeding. Additionally, treatment with a 600 mg loading dose of clopidogrel as compared to 300 mg (HR 0.49, p=0.01) did reduce acute and subacute ST, respectively. The question of whether higher doses of clopidogrel would improve cardiovascular outcomes was further evaluated in the CURRENT-OASIS 7 landmark trial in which 25,086 patients with ACS (29.2% STEMI) referred for an invasive strategy were randomized to double-dose clopidogrel (600 mg loading dose followed by 150 mg daily for six days and then 75 mg daily thereafter) versus standard dose (300 mg loading dose followed by 75 mg daily) [39, 40]. The investigators found that while there was no significant difference in the primary outcome of cardiovascular death, MI or stroke at 30 days in the overall population (4.2% in the double-dose group vs. 4.4% in the standard-dose group, p =0.30), double-dose clopidogrel was associated with a significant reduction in the rate of the primary outcome of cardiovascular death, MI or stroke at 30 days (3.9% vs. 4.5%, p =0.039) as well as in the rate of definite ST (0.7% vs. 1.3%, p=0.0001) in the prespecified subgroup of 17,263 patients who underwent PCI. Notably, major bleeding occurred slightly more frequently with the use of double-dose clopidogrel in both the overall group as well as the PCI subgroup (2.5% vs. 2.0%, p=0.01 and 1.6% vs. 1.1%, p=0.009, respectively). Several subsequent smaller studies including ISAR-CHOICE, ALBION, and PREPAIR have attempted to look at whether even higher loading doses of clopidogrel (900 mg and 1200 mg) might carry additional benefit when compared to the 600 mg and 300 mg doses [41–43]. These studies found that while treatment with increasing doses of clopidogrel did in fact result in greater levels of platelet inhibition, clinical endpoints such as MACE and troponin release were not statistically different. At this point, larger prospective trials evaluating clinical outcomes are needed before clopidogrel loading doses above 600 mg can be justified. With regards to the timing of double-dose clopidogrel pretreatment, the ISAR-REACT trial showed that among 2,159 patients undergoing PCI, a clopidogrel 600 mg loading dose could be given as early as two hours prior to PCI without detrimental effects when compared to longer durations of pre-treatment (2-3 hours, 3-6 hours, 6-12 hours, >12 hours) [44]. Similarly, the PRAGUE-8 and ARMYDA-5 PRELOAD trials reported no differences in outcomes when clopidogrel 600 mg was given to patients with stable angina or NSTE-ACS either before (mean of 19 and 6 hours respectively) or immediately after diagnostic coronary angiography, but prior to PCI [45, 46].

The RELOAD and ARMYDA-4 RELOAD trials attempted to address the question of whether an additional loading dose of clopidogrel was required prior to PCI in stable angina and ACS patients who were already receiving chronic clopidogrel therapy [47, 48]. The trials found that although clopidogrel reloading produced significantly greater levels of platelet inhibition, there was no difference in the primary endpoint of MACE. A subgroup analysis, however, showed that when reloaded with clopidogrel 600 mg, there was a significant benefit in patients with ACS who underwent PCI. While there is not enough evidence to make definitive recommendations regarding this issue, it may be reasonable to reload patients receiving chronic clopidogrel therapy with clopidogrel 600 mg prior to PCI for ACS or if their risk for ST is high.

## Prasugrel

Despite the increasing use of higher doses of clopidogrel, there are still many cases of breakthrough thrombotic events in patients who have undergone

PCI receiving standard DAPT [27]. Limitations of clopidogrel therapy have been attributed to its delayed onset of action, modest platelet inhibition effects, and a wide range of inter-individual variability with regards to platelet responsiveness given its dependence on the CYP system for prodrug metabolism. Prasugrel is a third-generation thienopyridine, and like clopidogrel also requires biotransformation to its active metabolite before irreversibly binding to $P2Y_{12}$ receptors and inhibiting platelet aggregation. In contrast to clopidogrel however, prasugrel has been shown to achieve greater levels of platelet inhibition more rapidly and more consistently among healthy individuals as well as in patients with CAD undergoing PCI [49, 50]. The JUMBO-TIMI 26 trial was a phase 2 randomized study of 904 patients designed to assess the safety of prasugrel when administered at the time of PCI and the results of this trial showed no difference in the rates of clinically significant bleeding events [51]. In the PRINCIPLE-TIMI 44 trial, 201 subjects were randomized to either prasugrel 60 mg or clopidogrel 600 mg as a loading dose one-half hour prior to elective PCI, and then to either prasugrel 10 mg or clopidogrel 150 mg as a maintenance dose [52]. The prasugrel groups achieved significantly greater levels of platelet inhibition in both the loading and maintenance phases. To assess prasugrel's clinical efficacy, the landmark TRITON-TIMI 38 trial enrolled 13,608 patients with moderate- to high-risk ACS (including both NSTE-ACS and STEMI) undergoing PCI and randomly assigned patients to either prasugrel (60 mg loading dose followed by 10 mg maintenance dose) or clopidogrel (300 mg loading dose followed by 75 mg maintenance dose) [53]. At 15-month follow-up, prasugrel reduced the composite endpoint of death, nonfatal MI or nonfatal stroke by 20% in comparison to clopidogrel (9.9% vs. 12.1%, HR 0.81, 95% CI 0.73-0.90, p<0.001) with the majority of the difference driven by lower rates of nonfatal MI (7.4% vs. 9.7%). ST, either definite or probable, was also significantly reduced with prasugrel compared to clopidogrel (1.1% vs. 2.4%, p<0.001) with similar outcomes between DES (0.84% vs. 2.31%) and BMS (1.27% vs. 2.41%) [54]. The risk for bleeding, however, was significantly increased in all categories including major bleeding (2.4% vs. 1.8%, p=0.03), life-threatening bleeding (1.4% vs. 0.9%, p=0.01), and fatal hemorrhage (0.4% vs. 0.1%, p=0.002). Risk factors for bleeding included age ≥75 years, history of stroke or TIA, and body weight <60 kg. When patients with these risk factors were excluded in a post-hoc analysis, the difference in bleeding rates became non-significant (HR 1.24, 95% CI 0.91 to 1.69, p=0.17) with prasugrel exhibiting even greater efficacy (HR 0.74, 95% CI 0.66 to 0.84, p<0.001). Additionally, the use of a GP IIb/IIIa inhibitor did not impact the relative risk of bleeding between patients treated with prasugrel as compared to clopidogrel [55]. Overall mortality did not differ significantly between the treatment groups.

## Ticragrelor

Ticragrelor is an oral antiplatelet agent from the cyclopentyl-triazolo-pyrimidine class that reversibly binds the ADP-P2Y$_{12}$ platelet receptor. Distinct from the thienopyridines, ticagrelor does not require metabolic conversion to its active form and is therefore not impacted by reduced bioavailability from hepatic prodrug conversion or competing CYP interactions [56]. Like prasugrel, it is known to produce a more rapid and intense reduction in platelet function when compared to clopidogrel and its reversible binding of the P2Y$_{12}$ receptor allows for more rapid washout of the antiplatelet effect. The ONSET/OFFSET study evaluated the antiplatelet effects of ticagrelor compared to clopidogrel in patients with stable CAD and found that ticagrelor achieved a more rapid and greater platelet inhibition than loading with high dose clopidogrel [57]. At two hours after loading, 98% of ticagrelor-treated patients were able to achieve >50% inhibition of platelets compared to only 31% of clopidogrel-treated patients (p<0.0001). Ticagrelor was also faster in offset, with the mean inhibition of platelet aggregation reduced to 58% by 24 hours after discontinuation. The 3- and 5-day inhibition of platelet aggregation for ticagrelor was equivalent to clopidogrel at days 5 and 7, respectively. Ticagrelor was also shown to achieve superior levels of platelet inhibition compared to prasugrel [32.9 P2Y$_{12}$ reaction units (PRU) vs. 101.3 PRU] in a randomized crossover study of ACS patients with high on-treatment platelet reactivity (OTR) on clopidogrel 24 hours after PCI [58].

In the landmark PLATO trial, 18,624 patients with ACS (38% STEMI) were randomized to either ticagrelor (180 mg loading dose followed by 90 mg twice daily) or clopidogrel (300 to 600 mg loading dose followed by 75 mg daily) in addition to chronic aspirin therapy [59]. At 12 months, treatment with ticagrelor was associated with a significant reduction in the primary efficacy endpoint of cardiovascular death, MI or stroke (9.8% vs. 11.7%, p<0.001) as well as the rate of all cause mortality (4.5% vs. 5.9%, p<0.001), MI alone, and ST. The reductions in ST for ticagrelor compared to clopidogrel were 1.6% vs. 2.4% (definite ST), 2.6% vs. 3.4% (definite or probable ST), and 3.3% vs. 4.3% (definite, probable, or possible ST). The anti-ischemic benefits of ticagrelor did come at a cost of increased major bleeding not related to CABG (4.5% vs. 3.8%, p=0.03), including more instances of fatal intracranial bleeds.

A subgroup analysis of patients with chronic kidney disease found that ticragrelor produced a more pronounced reduction in the primary endpoint when compared to patients with normal renal function as well as an overall decrease in total mortality [60]. An unexpected trend toward better outcomes was seen in the clopidogrel arm in North America leading investigators to hypothesize that the tendency to use higher doses of aspirin in North America offset the benefits of ticagrelor. One proposed mechanism links higher doses of aspirin with the inhibition of endogenous prostacyclin release, thereby shifting the influence of aspirin to a prothrombotic effect in the presence of strong $P2Y_{12}$ inhibition [61]. As such, the FDA issued a boxed warning that the use of ticagrelor with concurrent doses of aspirin over 100 mg daily would decrease the effectiveness of the drug.

## Recommendations for Antiplatelet Therapy in ACS

The 2009 ACC/AHA Joint STEMI/PCI updated guidelines provide recommendations for the choice of DAPT in patients with ACS in whom PCI is planned [62]. For all patients presenting with STEMI, aspirin should be administered as soon as possible. The choice for a second antiplatelet agent can include either clopidogrel (300 to 600 mg loading dose followed by 75 mg daily) [Class I, Level of Evidence C] or prasugrel (60 mg loading dose followed by 10 mg daily) [Class I, Level of Evidence B]. For STEMI patients who have received fibrinolytic therapy, clopidogrel at a loading dose of either 300 mg or 600 mg should be given followed by clopidogrel as the thienopyridine of choice for maintenance therapy [Class I, Level of Evidence C]. The choice and duration of maintenance therapy for ACS patients receiving a BMS or DES should be either clopidogrel 75 mg daily [Class I, Level of Evidence B] or prasugrel 10 mg daily (provided there are no contraindications) [Class I, Level of Evidence B] for at least 12 months unless the risk of morbidity due to bleeding outweighs the anticipated benefit of thienopyridine therapy, at which point earlier discontinuation should be considered [Class I, Level of Evidence C]. In patients in whom CABG is planned and can be delayed, it is recommended that clopidogrel be withdrawn for at least 5 days [Class I, Level of Evidence B] and prasugrel for at least 7 days [Class I, Level of Evidence C] unless the need for revascularization and/or the net benefit of the thienopyridine outweighs the risks of bleeding [Class I, Level of Evidence C]. Age $\geq 75$ years, history of TIA or stroke, and active major bleeding are contraindications to prasugrel therapy. Body weight

<60 kg is a relative contraindication to prasugrel therapy and consideration of lowering the maintenance dose from 10 mg to 5 mg daily should be given, though the safety and efficacy of the 5 mg dose have not been established.

The 2012 ACCF/AHA focused update of the guidelines for management of patients with UA/NSTEMI recommends that DAPT with aspirin plus a second antiplatelet agent be administered as early as possible to patients with definite UA/NSTEMI at medium or high risk in whom an early invasive strategy is planned [Class I, Level of Evidence A] [63]. If administered before PCI, the choice of a second antiplatelet agent to be added to aspirin can include one of the following: clopidogrel (600 mg loading dose followed by 75 mg daily thereafter) [Class I, Level of Evidence B], ticagrelor (180 mg loading dose followed by 90 mg twice daily) [Class I, Level of Evidence B], or alternatively an intravenous (IV) GP IIb/IIIa inhibitor [Class I, Level of Evidence B]. If administered at the time of PCI, the choice for a second antiplatelet agent to be added to aspirin can also include prasugrel (60 mg loading dose followed by 10 mg daily thereafter) [Class I, Level of Evidence B]. If both the risk for bleeding is low and the need for CABG is considered unlikely, prasugrel 60 mg may be considered for prompt administration upon presentation in patients with UA/NSTEMI for whom PCI is planned [Class IIb, Level of Evidence C]. Additionally, if the risk for bleeding is low, administration of clopidogrel at a loading dose of 600 mg followed by a higher maintenance dose of 150 mg daily for 6 days, then 75 mg daily thereafter may be reasonable [Class IIb, Level of Evidence B].

## Tailoring Antiplatelet Therapy Utilizing Platelet Function and Genetic Testing

Pharmacokinetic and pharmacodynamic data have revealed significant inter-individual variability in platelet response to clopidogrel, with reports of clopidogrel "hypo-responsiveness" in up to 30% of Caucasian patients. Patients with high (on treatment reactivity) OTR on clopidogrel have been shown to have worse cardiovascular outcomes and an increased incidence of ST after PCI [64, 65]. Utilizing the VerifyNow P2Y$_{12}$ assay (Accumetrics, San Diego), several trials have attempted to identify patients with high OTR who are considered low responders to clopidogrel in an effort to tailor antiplatelet therapy for the reduction of ST and other cardiovascular endpoints [66, 67]. In one study, over 1,600 patients undergoing DES implantation were treated with a 600 mg loading dose of clopidogrel and divided into quintiles based on their

OTR [68]. 323 patients, defined as low responders, were assigned to the upper quintile and found to have a significantly greater incidence of definite ST at 6 months compared to normal responders (2.5% vs. 0.4%, p<0.001), as well as a greater combined incidence of definite or probable ST over the same time period (4.1% vs. 0.7%, p<0.0001). The use of the VerifyNow P2Y$_{12}$ assay as a clinical guide for intensified platelet inhibition therapy was evaluated in the large multicenter trial, GRAVITAS, which randomized 2,214 patients undergoing PCI for stable CAD or NSTE-ACS with high OTR as defined by a PRU value of ≥230 to treatment with either double-dose clopidogrel (600 mg load followed by 150 mg daily for 6 months) or standard-dose clopidogrel (300 mg load followed by 75 mg daily for 6 months) [69]. Treatment with double-dose clopidogrel in patients with PRU≥230 failed to demonstrate a reduction in the primary endpoint of death, MI, or ST (2.3% vs. 2.3%, p=0.97) at 6 months, however a subsequent analysis found that achievement of OTR PRU<208 was associated with a lower risk for the primary endpoint at 60 days (HR 0.18, p=0.02) and 6 months (HR 0.43, p=0.01) [70]. A second trial, TRIGGER-PCI, compared the use of prasugrel versus clopidogrel in patients undergoing elective PCI with high OTR (defined as a lower PRU threshold of >208) [71]. Prasugrel was more effective at platelet inhibition than clopidogrel (median PRU decreased from a baseline of 245 to 80 at 3 months for prasugrel vs. 249 to 241 with clopidogrel, p<0.001), however, the trial was terminated early after enrolling only 423 patients out of a planned 2,150 due to an unexpected low rate of primary endpoint events (cardiovascular death or MI at 6 months), thus clinical conclusions could not be reached. This finding has led to great ambiguity in the interventional community with regards to tailoring individual antiplatelet therapy based on PRU levels alone, particularly in stable CAD patients.

Recent studies have focused on genetic variations in hepatic CYP isoenzymes as a potential cause of clopidogrel response variability, in particular single-nucleotide polymorphisms of CYP2C19. The GIFT study, a prespecified genetic substudy of GRAVITAS, identified an association of the reduced function CYP2C19*2 allele with persistently high OTR at 30 days and 6 months, irrespective of low- or high-dose clopidogrel therapy [72]. Additionally, a genetic substudy from TRITON-TIMI 38 found that patients with the reduced function CYP2C19*2 allele who were treated with clopidogrel had lower serum levels of active clopidogrel metabolite and diminished platelet inhibition leading to higher rates of ischemic events including ST when compared to non-carriers of the CYP2C19*2 allele (12.1% vs. 8.0%, HR 1.53, 95% CI 1.07 to 2.19, p = 0.01) [73]. A recent meta-analysis of over 42,000 patients, however, suggested that while an association between the CYP2C19 genotype and clopidogrel responsiveness exists, an association of genotype with cardiovascular events was not apparent [74].

It has been hypothesized that GRAVITAS and TRIGGER-PCI were negative trials because the patient population studied was at low risk for cardiovascular complications and ST (patients with stable CAD undergoing uncomplicated PCI using contemporary DES). Based on this, it may be argued that there is little role for platelet function testing in low risk patients and that it should be reserved for patients at higher risk for cardiovascular complications and ST, perhaps also targeting a lower PRU value of <208. The 2012 ACC/AHA guidelines for the management of UA/NSTEMI (or after ACS and PCI) include a Class IIb recommendation that platelet function testing or genotype assessment for a CYP2C19 loss of function variant might be considered if results of testing may alter management [63]. Whether a personalized approach to intensified platelet inhibition therapy can be beneficial in higher risk groups remains to be determined and will require further prospective investigation. As the role of platelet function testing in clinical practice continues to evolve, it is clear that certain subsets of patients with genetic predispositions, systemic disease processes, or unavoidable drug-drug interactions may have a reduced effectiveness of platelet inhibition with clopidogrel. In these groups of patients, many are not candidates for higher-dose clopidogrel or prasugrel therapy given the increased bleeding risk. To this end, novel antiplatelet agents that can reduce cardiovascular events and ST without an increase in bleeding complications remain a subject of ongoing investigations.

# Anti-Thrombotic Agents

## Unfractionated Heparin

Unfractionated heparin (UFH) inhibits platelet aggregation and fibrin formation by accelerating the action of antithrombin, which in turn inactivates factors IIa, IXa, and Xa. The evidence for UFH therapy in UA and NSTE-ACS has been well defined in early trials such as RISC and ATACS, [10, 12, 75–77] however, the benefits in acute STEMI are less clear. UFH use during PCI is believed to reduce the risk for acute vessel closure as well as catheter or wire thrombosis and has been extrapolated from data obtained from PTCA prior to the era of coronary stenting and DAPT [78]. Current ACC/AHA guidelines on the management of patients with STEMI recommend IV UFH therapy for all patients treated with a fibrin-specific fibrinolytic agent (alteplase, tenecteplase, reteplase) or a non-fibrin-specific agent (streptokinase, urokinase, anistreplase) if the risk for systemic embolization is high (large or anterior MI, atrial fibrillation, prior embolus, or known left ventricular thrombus). The goal for activated partial thromboplastin time (aPTT) should be 1.5-2.0 times control or between 50-70 seconds. The benefit of adjunctive UFH with fibrinolytic therapy is thought to be due to its effect on maintaining infarct vessel patency as there is limited data regarding any improvements in either mortality or reinfarction [79–82]. In patients with STEMI or UA/NSTEMI, it is recommended to continue UFH through the completion of uncomplicated PCI for those being referred for an invasive strategy. For those in whom medical therapy is planned, it is recommended to treat with UFH for at least 48 hours or until discharge [62, 63]. The most current ACC/AHA /SCAI guidelines for PCI recommend that in patients not receiving a GP IIb/IIIa inhibitor, UFH should be given using a bolus of 70-100 IU/kg to target an activated clotting time (ACT) between 250-350 seconds. For patients who are receiving a GP IIb/IIIa inhibitor, the heparin bolus should be lowered to 50-70 IU/kg to achieve an ACT of 200-250 seconds [83]. Heparin monitoring during PCI is generally done with ACT instead of aPTT as the anticoagulation levels required during the procedure are frequently too high for aPTT to track. An alternative strategy endorsed by the 2005 European Society of Cardiology guidelines for PCI is a single bolus of 100 IU/kg without ACT monitoring [84]. The routine use of UFH after uncomplicated procedures has not been shown to reduce ST and is not recommended given its association with increased rates of bleeding and vascular access complications. UFH use can cause autoimmune heparin-induced thrombocytopenia, a rare but potentially lethal complication associated with thrombosis. Treatment includes prompt withdrawal of all heparin products and initiation of alternative anticoagulation therapies (e.g., argatroban, lepirudin, bivalirudin).

## Low-Molecular-Weight Heparin

Like UFH, low-molecular-weight heparin (LMWH) prevents clot propagation but possesses several advantages over UFH due to different mechanisms of action. The ratio of anti-Xa/anti-IIa activity is significantly higher in LMWH compared to UFH, thereby inhibiting thrombin generation more effectively with potentially less bleeding. Suppression of the release of von Willebrand factor also augments LMWH's anticoagulant effect. Increased bioavailability leads to a longer duration of systemic anticoagulation and less binding to plasma proteins and produces a more consistent anticoagulant effect. Several trials including FRISC, FRIC, FRAXIS, TIMI 11-B, and ESSENCE have found that treatment with LMWH is at least as effective as UFH across a spectrum of ACS patients while maintaining a comparable safety profile [85–91]. The efficacy and safety of LMWH in PCI however is less certain. LMWH as compared to UFH was studied in 10,027 patients with NSTE-ACS being referred for early invasive strategy in the SYNERGY trial, and while enoxaparin use was shown to be non-inferior to UFH, it was associated with a significantly higher rate of major bleeding (9.1% vs. 7.6%) [92]. STEEPLE, a trial designed to assess the safety of enoxaparin (a single IV bolus of either 0.50 or 0.75 mg/kg prior to PCI) compared to UFH in 3,528 patients undergoing elective PCI was terminated early due to an excess mortality rate among the patients receiving lower dose enoxaparin [93]. As such, the 2005 ACC/AHA/SCAI guideline update for PCI recommends UFH as first line antithrombotic therapy in patients undergoing PCI except in patients with heparin-induced thrombocytopenia [Class I, Level of Evidence C]. LMWH is a reasonable alternative in patients with UA/NSTEMI [Class IIa, Level of Evidence B] and in patients with STEMI [Class IIb, Level of Evidence B] [83].

## Fondaparinux

Fondaparinux, a selective inhibitor of factor Xa, was tested against UFH in 350 patients undergoing urgent or elective PCI in the ASPIRE pilot trial and was found to have similar efficacy and safety outcomes [94]. This issue was further examined in the much larger OASIS-6 trial, which included 12,092 STEMI patients split into two strata based on whether UFH was indicated or not [95]. Stratum 1, in which UFH was not indicated, consisted of 5,658 patients, most of whom had received fibrinolytic therapy with streptokinase and in whom adequate reperfusion was achieved and PCI was not planned. Stratum 2 consisted of 6,434 patients in whom UFH was indicated (those who received a fibrin-specific fibrinolytic agent, those in whom adequate reperfusion was not achieved, or those in whom primary PCI was planned). Patients in each stratum were then randomized to receive either fondaparinux or placebo. Although there was an overall decrease in the primary endpoint of death or reinfarction with fondaparinux (9.7% vs. 11.2%), investigators found that this effect was driven mainly by a significant reduction in events in the stratum that did not receive heparin or primary PCI and that there was actually a trend towards worse outcomes with fondaparinux in the stratum of patients who received heparin and were treated with primary PCI. Fondaparinux use was also associated with a higher rate of catheter related thrombosis as well as coronary complications during PCI such as acute vessel closure, no reflow phenomenon, and dissection. Therefore, the 2007 focused update of the ACC/AHA/SCAI guidelines for PCI do not recommend fondaparinux use as the sole anticoagulant to support PCI and when used should be supplemented with another agent that has anti-IIa activity such as UFH or bivalirudin [96].

## Direct Thrombin Inhibitors

Direct thrombin inhibitors (e.g., hirudin, bivalirudin, lepirudin) inactivate thrombin by binding directly to its catalytic site and hold several advantages over UFH in that antithrombin is not required as a cofactor allowing clot-bound thrombin to be inactivated [97]. Additionally, there is no thrombin-mediated activation of platelets. Hirudin, a naturally occurring peptide derived from the saliva of the medicinal leech has been studied in patients with ACS undergoing reperfusion therapy with fibrinolytics or PCI (TIMI-9B, GUSTO-IIB, HELVETICA) and found to have no benefit when compared to UFH with comparable rates of major bleeding [98–100]. The pilot trial HERO reproduced a similar finding with bivalirudin, a synthetic peptide that directly inhibits free and clot-bound thrombin [101]. When given concurrently with streptokinase, bivalirudin was more effective than UFH in producing early infarct-related artery patency (TIMI grade 3 flow) without increasing the risk of major bleeding. The follow up HERO-2 mortality trial found that bivalirudin had similar rates of mortality at 30 days (10.5% vs. 10.9% with UFH, OR 0.99) with a small reduction in reinfarction at 96 hours (1.6% vs. 2.3%) and a non-significant trend toward more severe bleeding (0.6% vs. 0.4%) [102].

The role of bivalirudin in primary PCI was evaluated in the HORIZONS-AMI trial in which 3,602 patients with STEMI undergoing primary PCI were randomized to receive treatment with either UFH plus a GP IIb/IIIa inhibitor or to treatment with bivalirudin alone with provisional GP IIb/IIIa inhibitor [103]. The investigators found that anticoagulation with bivalirudin alone resulted in lower rates of MACE at 30 days (9.2% vs. 12.1%, RR 0.76, 95%

CI 0.63-0.92, p=0.005), major bleeding (4.9% vs. 8.3%, RR 0.60, 95% CI 0.46-0.77, p<0.001), 30-day death from cardiac causes (1.8% vs. 2.9%, RR 0.62, 95% CI 0.40-0.95, p=0.03), and 30-day overall mortality (2.1% vs. 3.1%, RR 0.66, 95% CI 0.44-1.00, p=0.047). There was a concern about a significant 1% increase in acute ST seen within 24 hours, however the rates for ST at 30 days were similar in both groups. Bivalirudin was further examined in the REPLACE-2, ISAR-REACT 3, and ACUITY randomized trials evaluating patients across a broad spectrum of disease (stable CAD to high-risk ACS) undergoing PCI [104–106]. The results of these trials solidified bivalirudin's favorable safety and efficacy profile when compared to UFH plus a GP IIb/IIIa inhibitor by demonstrating non-inferiority for preventing ischemic complications after PCI along with a reduction in rates of major bleeding. Additionally, a meta-analysis of randomized trials revealed that bivalirudin use provided greater absolute benefits in the prevention of ischemic and bleeding complications in patients with renal insufficiency [107]. The 2009 AHA/ACC joint STEMI/PCI focused update recommendations state that bivalirudin is a useful supportive measure for primary PCI with or without prior treatment with UFH [Class I, Level of Evidence B]. Additionally, for patients with STEMI undergoing PCI who are at high risk for bleeding, bivalirudin anticoagulation is a reasonable choice [Class IIa, Level of Evidence B] [62].

## Glycoprotein IIb/IIIa Inhibitors

GP IIb/IIIa is an integrin receptor expressed on the surface membrane of platelets that undergoes a conformational change following platelet activation allowing it to bind to fibrinogen and cross-link with other platelets. This forms the basis for platelet aggregation and the pathologic vascular thrombosis seen in ACS. Three GP IIb/IIIa inhibitors are currently approved for use in ACS and PCI although much of the evidence supporting their use was established in the era prior to standard DAPT.

Abciximab is the Fab fragment of a human-murine monoclonal antibody directed at the GP IIb/IIIa receptor. A number of clinical trials have attempted to evaluate its use in patients undergoing PCI for stable angina or ACS. These include EPIC, EPILOG, CAPTURE, RAPPORT, ADMIRAL, ISAR-2, ISAR-REACT, ISAR-SWEET, CADILLAC, ACE, EPISTENT, and ERASER [108–119]. Pooled analyses of several of these trials have found that abciximab significantly reduced the incidence of 30-day death and MI when compared to placebo (HR 0.55, 95% CI 0.43-0.69, p<0.001) [120]. This benefit was found regardless of the type of coronary intervention used including balloon angioplasty, elective stenting, bailout stenting, and directional atherectomy, without an increase in significant bleeding complications. Protection from major adverse outcomes with abciximab continued out to six months and was independent of gender and a significant mortality benefit persisted at three years (6.4% vs. 5.0%, HR 0.78, 95% CI 0.63-0.98, p=0.03) [121, 122]. In the BRAVE-3 study, 800 patients presenting within 24 hours of STEMI were treated with aspirin, clopidogrel 600 mg, and randomized to either abciximab or placebo given prior to primary PCI [123]. There were no significant differences between the two groups with respect to the primary endpoint of infarct size as measured by single-photon emission computed tomography or in 30-day MACE.

Tirofiban is a non-peptide molecule that exhibits dose-dependent inhibition of the GP IIb/IIIa receptor. The RESTORE trial randomized 2,139 patients with ACS undergoing PTCA with balloon angioplasty or directional atherectomy to either placebo or tirofiban (10 μg/kg/3 min IV bolus followed by continuous infusion of 0.15 μg/kg/min for 36 hours) [124]. The composite end point (death from any cause, MI, bypass surgery for angioplasty failure or recurrent ischemia necessitating repeat PCI) was reduced by tirofiban at two days (RR 38%, p<0.005) and at seven days (RR 27%, p=0.022) post-PTCA, however this reduction was no longer statistically significant at 30 days (10.3% vs. 12.2%, p=0.16) and at 6-month follow-up [125]. The ADVANCE trial then evaluated whether higher doses of tirofiban would confer a benefit in 202 patients with ACS undergoing primary PCI [126]. Patients were randomly assigned to either placebo or tirofiban (25 μg/kg/3 min bolus plus 0.15 μg/kg/min continuous infusion for 24-48 hours). The results of this study showed that treatment with high dose tirofiban produced a significant reduction in the primary endpoint of death, MI, TVR, or bailout use of a GP IIb/IIIa inhibitor (35% vs. 20%, HR 0.51, 95% CI 0.29-0.88, p=0.01). The difference was driven by a reduction in MI and bailout use of GP IIb/IIIa inhibitors with no significant effect on mortality. Bleeding rates were comparable between tirofiban and placebo. Subgroup analyses found that while patients with ACS benefitted from tirofiban use, those with stable angina did not. Diabetics also appeared to gain a benefit with tirofiban while non-diabetics did not. Upstream use of tirofiban prior to PCI in patients with STEMI was evaluated in three trials: TIGER-PA, ON-TIME, and ON-TIME 2 [127–129]. These trials demonstrated that tirofiban use was generally associated with improved electrocardiographic endpoints such as resolution of ST-segment elevations with no increase in the risk of major or minor bleeding.

In the ON-TIME 2 trial, 984 patients with STEMI were randomized to pretreatment with either high dose tirofiban or placebo prior to PCI and while there was an improvement in ST-segment resolution in the tirofiban group, there was no significant difference between the two groups in angiographic variables such as TIMI grade 3 flow or blush grade. Later results from ON-TIME 2 however reported a significant reduction in 30-day MACE in the tirofiban group (5.8% vs. 8.6%, p=0.043) that was maintained at 1-year follow-up (3.7% vs. 5.8%, p=0.08) [130].

Eptifibatide is a synthetic, non-immunogenic cyclic heptapeptide inhibitor of GP IIb/IIIa with an active pharmacophore, which is derived from the structure of barbourin, a GP IIb/IIIa inhibitor isolated from the venom of the Southeastern pigmy rattlesnake [131]. It has a rapid onset of action with a plasma half-life of 10-15 minutes making its antiplatelet effect rapidly reversible. Its use in ACS and PCI has been evaluated in several clinical trials including the PURSUIT trial, in which 10,948 patients were randomized to eptifibatide or placebo in conjunction with UFH and aspirin [132]. By four days, the combined endpoint of death and nonfatal MI were reduced by 1.5% in the eptifibatide group (14.2% vs. 15.7%, p=0.04). More remarkably, this benefit was apparent as early as 96 hours and persisted through 30 days with a greater benefit observed in patients undergoing early angioplasty [133]. In the IMPACT-II trial of 4,010 patients undergoing elective, urgent or emergent PCI, treatment with eptifibatide during PCI reduced the rates of early abrupt vessel closure and ischemic events by 30 days [134]. The benefits of eptifibatide have also been shown in patients undergoing elective PCI, as seen in the ESPRIT trial that randomized 2,064 patients to pretreatment with placebo or eptifibatide prior to PCI [135]. The trial was terminated early for efficacy as pretreatment with ebtifibatide led to a significant reduction in the primary end point of death, MI, urgent revascularization, or need for bailout GP IIb/IIIa inhibitor at 48 hours (6.6% vs. 10.5%, p=0.0015) as well as at 30 days (6.8% vs. 10.5%, p=0.0034). With regards to safety endpoints, bleeding rates with eptifibatide were equivalent to placebo in IMPACT-II (4.8% vs. 5.1%), although severe bleeding without hemorrhagic stroke was increased in PURSUIT (11.6% vs. 9.2%). Additionally, a pooled analysis of eight randomized control trials showed that eptifibatide did not significantly increase the rate of thrombocytopenia compared to placebo [136].

The general benefits of IV GP IIb/IIIa inhibitors were evaluated in a meta-analysis pooling data from 21 trials involving patients with a broad range of CAD [137]. The study reported that GP IIb/IIIa inhibitor use produced significant reductions in the combined end point of 30-day death, MI, or urgent revascularization in patients undergoing PCI (7.8% vs. 11.6%), in patients with NSTE-ACS (11.4% vs. 12.8%), and in patients with acute STEMI who underwent angioplasty (3.9% vs. 7.8%). The benefits of adjunctive GP IIb/IIIa inhibitors in acute STEMI remain uncertain however. As discussed in the section on bivalirudin, the HORIZONS-AMI trial randomized 3,602 patients with STEMI undergoing primary PCI to UFH with a GP IIb/IIIa inhibitor (either abciximab or eptifibatide) or to bivalirudin alone with provisional GP IIb/IIIa [103]. All patients were treated with aspirin and a thienopyridine prior to PCI. Of the 1,661 patients who were randomized to treatment with UFH, 757 received a double bolus of eptifibatide and 863 received abciximab. In the bivalirudin alone plus provisional GP IIb/IIIa arm, only 53 of 1,674 patients received eptifibatide and 72 received abciximab. At 30 days, the primary endpoint of MACE as well as major bleeding was higher in the group that received UFH and a GP IIb/IIIa inhibitor as compared to bivalirudin alone. A subgroup analysis of the UFH plus GP IIb/IIIa group compared those treated with eptifibatide and abciximab and found that there was no significant difference in the incidence of ST at one year [138].

With regards to the timing of adjunctive GP IIb/IIIa use in patients undergoing PCI for acute STEMI, a meta-analysis of six randomized trials including TIGER-PA and ON-TIME, found that early administration (prior to transfer to catheterization laboratory) as compared to late (at the time of PCI) improved measures of coronary patency as well as clinical outcomes [139]. The FINESSE trial also addressed the issue of timing of GP IIb/IIIa inhibitor therapy. In the trial, 2,453 patients with STEMI were randomized to pre-PCI treatment with a half-dose fibrinolytic agent plus abciximab, pre-PCI abciximab alone, or abciximab at the time of PCI [140]. The primary endpoint was composite death, ventricular fibrillation occurring over 48 hours after randomization, cardiogenic shock and congestive heart failure during the first 90 days after randomization. The results of this trial showed no benefit and perhaps a trend towards more bleeding with abciximab pretreatment as compared to abciximab given at the time of PCI.

With regards to its safety profile, there does appear to be an increased risk of bleeding with the use of IV GP IIb/IIIa inhibitors, however a pooled analysis of 14 randomized trials including approximately 28,000 patients found no difference in the incidence of intracerebral hemorrhage when comparing heparin plus any GP IIb/IIIa inhibitor to heparin plus placebo (0.12% vs. 0.09%, OR 1.3), or when comparing a GP IIb/IIIa inhibitor alone with heparin alone [141].

When deciding between agents for use in PCI, it is unclear whether one GP IIb/IIIa inhibitor holds any significant advantage in clinical efficacy over another. It is likely that the level of platelet inhibition achieved at two hours is similar between all three agents although there is some suggestion that the current recommended dosing regimen for tirofiban produces relatively less platelet inhibition in the first 15-60 minutes after coronary intervention [142]. One of the few clinical trials to compare the clinical efficacy of two GP IIb/IIIa inhibitors head-to-head was the TARGET trial in which 4,809 patients undergoing elective PCI were randomly assigned to either abciximab or tirofiban [143]. The study showed that abciximab (0.25 mg/kg bolus followed by 0.125 µg/kg [maximum 10 µg/min] for 12 hours) was significantly superior to tirofiban (10 µg/kg bolus followed by 0.15 µg/kg for 18-24 hours) in reducing the composite endpoint of death, MI, or urgent revascularization at 30 days (6% vs. 7.6%, HR 0.79). The difference appeared to be driven mainly by less procedure related MIs in the abciximab group (5.4% vs. 6.9%). A subgroup analysis found that this benefit was limited to patients who had ACS or were non-diabetic. At six months however, there was no longer any difference in the primary composite endpoint between the two drugs and by one year, the benefit of abciximab in the subgroup of patients with ACS had disappeared [144,145]. A higher tirofiban bolus dose regimen (25 µg/kg bolus over three minutes followed by 0.15 µg/kg/min for 18 hours) given prior to PCI was to be compared with pretreatment with abciximab in the TENACITY trial, however the trial was halted due to insufficient funding. MULTISTRATEGY was an open-label, multi-center European trial, which randomized 745 patients with STEMI undergoing primary PCI in a 2-by-2 factorial design to pretreatment with either high-dose tirofiban or abciximab and sirolimus-eluting stent versus BMS [146]. All patients received standard DAPT with aspirin and clopidogrel as well as systemic anticoagulation with UFH. There was no significant difference between the GP IIb/IIIa groups in the primary end points of ST-segment resolution at 90 minutes after PCI (RR 1.020, 95% CI 0.958-1.086, p=0.001 for non-inferiority) and the rate of MACE at 8 months. Rates of major and minor bleeding complications were similar, however the incidence of moderate or severe thrombocytopenia was increased with abciximab (4.0% vs. 0.8%, p=0.004). To date abciximab has not been directly compared to ebtifibatide to evaluate relative clinical efficacy, although one study showed that compared to tirofiban, ebtifibatide was as effective as abciximab in achieving a greater proportion of patients in whom there was greater than 80% inhibition of platelet activation at 15 minutes [142]. A retrospective analysis of 452 patients with STEMI undergoing primary PCI who received adjunctive therapy with either abciximab or eptifibatide found no significant differences in clinical outcomes including reinfarction (2% vs. 3% for eptifibatide and abciximab respectively), repeat revascularization (3% vs. 4%), bleeding complications (8% vs. 12%), congestive heart failure (5% vs. 3%), cerebrovascular accidents (0% vs. 2%), renal failure (2% vs. 3%), and all-cause mortality at discharge (5% vs. 4%) as well as at 6 months (6.5% vs. 6.4%, HR 0.976, 95% CI 0.43-2.23, log-rank, p=0.95) [147].

Given the above evidence, the 2009 AHA/ACC joint STEMI/PCI focused update recommendations concluded that in the setting of DAPT with aspirin and a thienopyridine plus either UFH or bivalirudin as the anticoagulant, GP IIb/IIIa inhibitors can be useful at the time of primary PCI but cannot be recommended as routine therapy. In select cases such as for the patient with a large thrombus burden or for patients who have not received adequate thienopyridine loading, adjunctive treatment with a GP IIb/IIIa inhibitor (abciximab [Class IIa, Level of Evidence A], tirofiban [Class IIa, Level of Evidence B], or eptifibatide [Class IIa, Level of Evidence B]) may be of more benefit [62].

## Fibrinolytic Therapy

Fibrinolytic therapy restores blood flow in the infarct-related artery and has been shown to improve mortality in STEMI patients who are not able to receive timely PCI, though not in patients with NSTE-ACS. The mortality benefit of fibrinolytic therapy was first demonstrated with streptokinase in the GISSI-2 and ISIS-2 landmark trials [11, 148–151]. Streptokinase is a single chain polypeptide derived from beta-hemolytic streptococcus that binds to and cleaves peptide bonds on plasminogen causing an indirect conformational change that then activates plasmin. Streptokinase is antigenic and can infrequently cause an immunologic sensitization and allergic reaction with repeated use exposure. Increased doses are required to neutralize the body's anti-streptococcal antibodies.

Alteplase (recombinant tissue-type plasminogen activator, t-PA) is a serine protease that is naturally produced by endothelial cells and possesses no antigenic features. In contrast to streptokinase (non-fibrin specific), t-PA is one of several fibrin-specific agents whose ability to convert plasminogen to plasmin is greatly enhanced after binding preferentially to fibrin in a thrombus with resultant local fibrinolysis. The results of the clinical trial GUSTO-I comparing streptokinase and t-PA in 41,021 patients with STEMI demonstrated an absolute survival benefit of 1% with t-PA at 30 days (6.3% vs. 7.3%) that persisted at one year (9.1% vs. 10.1%) with the most benefit seen in patients less than 75 years old and in those with anterior wall infarctions [82, 152]. Streptokinase, however, remains the most widely used fibrinolytic agent worldwide. Although it is less efficacious than alteplase, it maintains a reasonable efficacy to safety ratio with a lower risk of intra-cranial hemorrhage and is significantly less expensive.

Two other genetically engineered fibrin-specific agents currently approved in the US for use in the treatment of acute STEMI include reteplase (r-PA) and tenecteplase (TNK). Like t-PA, these agents are not antigenic and have no associated risk of allergic reaction. r-PA is a recombinant nonglycosylated form of human tissue plasminogen activator. In comparison to t-PA, r-PA has a longer half-life and binds fibrin with lower affinity improving its ability to penetrate into clots, though clinical trials (RAPID I and II, GUSTO III, INJECT) have generally demonstrated similar outcomes with r-PA and t-PA [153–157]. The newest of these, tenecteplase (TNK) is a recombinant plasminogen activator derived from the native t-PA. It possesses 14 times more specificity to fibrin and is 80 times more resistant to inhibition by plasminogen activator inhibitor-1 [158]. It has a longer plasma half-life, allowing for easier and faster treatment with a single IV bolus injection and has been shown in several clinical trials including TIMI 10A and 10B, ASSENT-1 and ASSENT-2, to be as effective as t-PA with a significant reduction in non-cerebral bleeding [159–162].

Lanoteplase (n-PA) is another genetically engineered mutant of wild-type t-PA, however, it is not currently approved for use due to an increase in hemorrhagic stroke [163, 164]. Anistreplase (APSAC) is another fibrinolytic agent that has a significantly longer half-life compared to streptokinase (90-100 minutes vs. 18-23 minutes). Like streptokinase and staphylokinase, it is antigenic leading to restrictions in repeated use. Though its efficacy and safety profiles were similar to streptokinase, anistreplase is no longer available. Urokinase is a non-fibrin specific fibrinolytic and is a nonselective activator of plasminogen. Urokinase is currently used only in the treatment of pulmonary embolism.

Absolute contraindications to fibrinolytic therapy include any history of intracranial hemorrhage, history of ischemic stroke within the preceding three months, presence of a cerebral vascular malformation or a primary or metastatic intracranial malignancy, symptoms or signs suggestive of an aortic dissection, a bleeding diathesis or active bleeding with the exception of menses, and a significant closed-head trauma within the preceding three months [62]. Furthermore, combination therapy with fibrinolytic agents and GP IIb/IIIa inhibitors is not recommended owing to a lack of mortality benefit with significantly higher rates of bleeding seen in the GUSTO V and ASSENT-3 trials [165–170].

In patients with acute STEMI, PCI has been shown to be more effective than fibrinolytic therapy in preventing death, reinfarction, and stroke [171]. However, many patients are unable to receive prompt PCI, particularly those who first present to a hospital without PCI capabilities. In such cases, it is recommended that patients who are eligible receive early fibrinolytic therapy. The issue of whether and when to perform coronary angiography and PCI in patients who have received fibrinolytic therapy is complex and has been examined extensively in clinical trials. Evidence suggests that patients who are able to attain normalization of blood flow (TIMI grade 3) in the infarct-related artery after fibrinolysis tend to have the most favorable outcomes [82, 172]. Although fibrinolytic therapy restores patency (TIMI grade 2 or 3) in 80% of infarct-related arteries, it only restores normalization of flow (TIMI grade 3) in 50-60% of arteries. This provides the rationale for performing PCI following the administration of fibrinolytic therapy. Two trials, GRACIA-2 and FAST-MI, have demonstrated equivalency in efficacy and safety when comparing fibrinolytic therapy followed by PCI to primary PCI [173, 174]. Previously used terms describing specific reperfusion strategies with PCI after fibrinolytic therapy have included *facilitated PCI* and *rescue PCI*, however, the 2009 ACC/AHA joint STEMI/PCI focused update considered these labels potentially misleading. Though these terms are no longer used in the recommendations, many of the previous supporting trials refer to these strategies so a brief review will be necessary.

Facilitated PCI involves initial treatment with full or half dose fibrinolytic agent or a combination of fibrinolytic and GP IIb/IIIa agents followed by immediate PCI. Two large, randomized clinical trials have addressed this issue. The trial ASSENT-4-PCI was intended to randomize 4,000 patients with STEMI who presented within 6 hours of symptom onset to full-dose tenecteplase or placebo prior to primary PCI [175]. The trial was terminated early due to a significant increase in the primary endpoint of death, heart failure, or shock within 90 days in the tenecteplase group (19% vs. 13%, RR 1.39, 95% CI 1.11-1.74), along with increased mortality (6% vs. 3%), in-hospital stroke (1.8% vs. 0%; mostly intracranial hemorrhage), as well as reinfarction (6% vs. 4%) and TVR (7% vs. 3%) at 90 days. The FINESSE trial, described in more detail in the GP IIb/IIIa section, showed that there was no benefit in the treatment of acute STEMI with half-dose reteplase and abciximab prior to PCI with trends toward an increase in intracranial hemorrhage as well as major and minor bleeding [140]. One possible explanation for the poor outcomes seen with facilitated PCI is the immediate nature of planned PCI after fibrinolytic therapy (median time period of 104 minutes between tenecteplase and PCI in the ASSENT-4- PCI trial). Recanalization of the infarct artery occurs 30-45 minutes after tenecteplase injection, so the relatively short time gain from the point of recanalization until PCI likely exposes the patient to more bleeding risk associated with full-dose fibrinolytic and antithrombotic therapy relative to any potential smaller benefit of PCI. A subgroup analysis showing a trend toward better outcomes when tenecteplase was given in the ambulance compared to much worse outcomes when given at a PCI center is consistent with this theory. The results of these and various smaller trials, as well as a 2006 meta-analysis have led most major society guidelines to recommend against facilitated PCI with full dose fibrinolytic therapy, though the 2007 ACC/AHA/SCAI focused update of guidelines for PCI makes a weak recommendation for the consideration of facilitated PCI using regimens other than full-dose fibrinolytic therapy in patients with high-risk STEMI in whom bleeding risk is low and PCI is not immediately available within 90 minutes [Class IIb, Level of Evidence C] [96].

Rescue PCI refers to the strategy of performing PCI only if there are clinical or electrocardiographic signs of failed reperfusion of the infarct artery after treatment with fibrinolytics. The 2007 ACC/AHA/SCAI focused update of guidelines for PCI make strong recommendations for rescue PCI or emergency CABG for cardiogenic shock in patients less than 75 years of age [Class I, Level of Evidence B], severe congestive heart failure and/or pulmonary edema (Killip class III) [Class I, Level of Evidence B], or hemodynamically compromising ventricular arrhythmias [Class I, Level of Evidence C]. Rescue PCI is also reasonable for cardiogenic shock in patients 75 years of age or older if they are suitable candidates for revascularization, hemodynamic or electrical instability, persistent ischemic symptoms, or for <50% ST-segment resolution in the lead that showed the greatest degree of ST elevation at presentation at 90 minutes after initiation of fibrinolytic therapy and a moderate or large area of myocardium at risk (anterior MI, inferior MI with right ventricular involvement or precordial ST-segment depression). These recommendations were based largely on results from the REACT trial as well as a subsequent meta-analysis of 8 rescue PCI trials demonstrating a clear benefit of rescue PCI over repeated doses of fibrinolytic therapy or medical management for failed fibrinolysis [176–179].

As stated above, the most current ACC/AHA guidelines for STEMI/PCI have abandoned the potentially confusing terms facilitated PCI (immediate planned PCI usually performed within 2 hours of fibrinolytic or fibrinolytic plus GP IIb/IIIa therapy) and rescue PCI (PCI reserved for only those who fail fibrinolysis) in favor of a *pharmacoinvasive strategy*. Several trials have provided valuable evidence informing the guidelines on this matter. In the CARESS-in-AMI trial, 600 STEMI patients 75 years of age or younger with one or more high-risk features (extensive ST-segment elevation, new left bundle branch block, previous MI, Killip class >2, or left ventricular ejection fraction ≤35%) were treated with half-dose reteplase, abciximab, heparin, and aspirin, and randomly assigned to immediate transfer for PCI or to standard medical management at the local hospital with transfer only for rescue PCI. [180].

The primary outcome was a composite of death, reinfarction, or refractory ischemia at 30 days. PCI was performed in 85.6% of the patients assigned to immediate transfer for PCI and rescue PCI was performed in 30.3% of the standard care/rescue PCI group. The primary outcome occurred significantly less in the immediate PCI group compared to standard care/rescue PCI (4.4% vs. 10.7%, HR 0.40, 95% CI 0.21-0.76, log rank p=0.004). There was no difference in major bleeding or strokes between the two groups. In the TRANSFER-AMI trial, 1,059 high-risk STEMI patients who were treated with tenecteplase within two hours of symptom onset were then randomized to either immediate transfer for cardiac catheterization (PCI within 6 hours) or to standard medical care [181]. High-risk STEMI was defined as ST-segment elevation ≥2 mm in two anterior leads or ST-segment elevation ≥1 mm in two inferior leads plus one or more of the following: systolic blood pressure <100 mmHg, heart rate >100 beats/min, Killip class II or III, ST-segment depression ≥2 mm in the anterior leads, or ST-segment ≥1 mm in one right sided lead (V4R). Standard care included rescue PCI if required or delayed angiography >24 hours after STEMI. All patients received aspirin, tenecteplase, and heparin or enoxaparin with a recommendation for clopidogrel.

The primary endpoint was the composite of death, reinfarction, recurrent ischemia, new or worsening congestive heart failure, or cardiogenic shock within 30 days. Cardiac catheterization PCI were performed in 98.5% and 84.9% of the patients assigned to early PCI at a median of 2.8 hours after randomization and in 88.7% and 67.4% of the patients assigned to standard treatment at a median of 32.5 hours after randomization.

At 30 days, the primary endpoint occurred was significantly reduced in the early PCI group (11.0% vs. 17.2%, RR 0.64, 95% CI 0.47-0.87, p=0.004) with no significant differences between the groups in the incidence of major bleeding. Several other trials have evaluated the timing of PCI after fibrinolysis with an early pharmacoinvasive therapy compared to standard care including GRACIA-1, NORDISTEMI, and SIAM III [182–184].

Each had a different study design and thus examined slightly different patient populations but all have confirmed the observations seen in CARESS-in-AMI and TRANSFER-AMI that a pharmacoinvasive strategy with immediate or early PCI after fibrinolytic therapy (within 3-24 hours) produces better outcomes than standard medical care with rescue PCI or routine late PCI (over 24 hours).

Based on the above evidence, a pharmacoinvasive approach to the management of STEMI patients who present to a hospital without PCI capabilities has been developed, which includes routine use of a pharmacologic agent (either fibrinolytic therapy or a GP IIb/IIIa inhibitor) prior to transfer to a PCI-capable hospital for diagnostic angiogram and consideration of PCI. Patients with STEMI who present to a PCI capable hospital are not recommended to receive fibrinolytic therapy and should undergo prompt PCI no later than 90 minutes after presentation. STEMI patients who present to a hospital without PCI capability should be triaged to either immediate transfer for PCI or to receive fibrinolytic therapy if deemed an appropriate candidate.

Those with high-risk STEMI features (congestive heart failure, cardiogenic shock, electrical instability, etc.), elevated bleeding risk with fibrinolytic therapy, or presenting more than 4 hours after symptom onset may be better suited for immediate transfer for PCI without delay for fibrinolytic therapy if the time required for transport to the receiving hospital is not prolonged. STEMI patients who present early after symptom onset with low bleeding risk are the most suitable candidates for fibrinolytic therapy. If after receiving the fibrinolytic agent the patient is deemed to have high-risk features, the patient should then be immediately transferred for PCI with the intention to perform diagnostic catheterization with possible PCI within 3-24 hours of presentation. Patients who are not judged to be high-risk may be transferred to a PCI-capable hospital after receiving antithrombotic therapy or may be observed in the initial facility.

# Novel Agents

## Cangrelor

Like ticagrelor, cangrelor is a reversible, non-thienopyridine antagonist of the ADP-P2Y$_{12}$ receptor, though it differs in its IV route of administration, which allows it to achieve a rapid onset and offset of action. Cangrelor is an adenosine triphosphate analog that is metabolized via dephosphorylation pathways and has a plasma half-life of 3-6 minutes resulting in return of normal platelet function within 30-60 minutes after discontinuation of cangrelor. Similar to the GP IIb/IIIa inhibitor abciximab, cangrelor exhibits a dose-dependent inhibition of platelets, though with less bleeding time prolongation and a faster normalization of platelet function [185]. CHAMPION PCI and CHAMPION PLATFORM were large trials that randomized high-risk patients (>50% NSTEMI) undergoing PCI to treatment with cangrelor (IV bolus and infusion) plus a 600 mg loading dose of clopidogrel versus placebo plus clopidogrel [186, 187]. The major difference between the two trials was the timing of study drug administration. Patients in CHAMPION PCI received both drugs within 30 minutes before PCI while patients in CHAMPION PLATFORM received cangrelor prior to PCI and clopidogrel only after completion of PCI. Both trials were terminated early due to a lack of significant difference in the primary composite endpoint of death from any cause, MI, or ischemia-driven revascularization at 48 hours (7.5% vs. 7.1% for placebo, p=0.59, in CHAMPION PCI) and (7.0% vs. 8.0% for placebo, p=0.17, in CHAMPION PLATFORM). Two prespecified secondary endpoints, death and ST at 48 hours, did not differ between treatment groups in CHAMPION PCI (ST rates of 0.2% vs. 0.3% for placebo, p=0.34), though in CHAMPION PLATFORM, both were found to be significantly lower in the cangrelor group compared to placebo (ST occurred in 5 vs. 16 patients for placebo, 0.2% vs. 0.6%, OR 0.31, 95% CI 0.11 to 0.85, p=0.02) with the differences remaining significant at 30 days. The authors of the study noted however, that since the primary endpoint of the trial was negative, any interpretation of secondary endpoints must be made with caution and should only serve as hypothesis generating. A third large randomized trial comparing cangrelor and clopidogrel standard therapy (CHAMPION PHOENIX) is currently underway, enrolling patients with predominantly ACS who are P2Y$_{12}$ inhibitor naive and will include ST in their primary composite endpoint [188].

As both cangrelor and clopidogrel competitively bind the ADP-P2Y$_{12}$ receptor, a follow up platelet substudy using patient data from the two CHAMPION trials was performed to evaluate whether any pharmacodynamic interaction existed between the drugs that may have limited cangrelor's efficacy in the trials [189]. Although platelet inhibition was significantly greater with cangrelor infusion (11% of patients treated with cangrelor plus clopidogrel had PRU>235 compared to 69% with clopidogrel alone, p<0.001), there was no significant difference in the primary endpoint of achieving <20% change in PRU from baseline to >10 hours after the end of infusion (38.1% vs. 25.3%, p=0.076). Overall, these findings confirm the more rapid and potent platelet inhibition of cangrelor as compared to clopidogrel, though the combination of the two drugs does not appear to add to or detract from platelet inhibitory effects. While these data do not suggest the presence of a pharmacodynamic interaction between cangrelor and clopidogrel, further investigations are needed to elucidate any potential interaction.

The BRIDGE study was a small trial that included 210 post-PCI or ACS patients who required cessation of thienopyridine therapy prior to scheduled CABG [190]. Patients were randomized to either cangrelor infusion (0.75 μg/kg/min IV) or placebo for at least 48 hours. The results showed that patients treated with cangrelor had significantly lower levels of platelet reactivity (PRU<240) as compared to placebo (98.8% vs. 19.0%, p=0.001) with no significant increase in major bleeding prior to CABG. While cangrelor is not yet commercially available, it may become a valuable tool in the future to help fill an important niche role in patients at risk for cardiac events or ST while awaiting surgery.

## Cilostazol

Cilostazol inhibits phosphodiesterase III, which leads to increased cyclic AMP, resulting in vasodilation as well as a reversible inhibition of platelet aggregation, vascular smooth muscle cell proliferation and neointimal hyperplasia. It has been approved for the treatment of intermittent claudication in patients with peripheral vascular disease and is contraindicated in patients with heart failure of any severity due to an increased risk of death. Several studies have found that the addition of cilostazol to traditional DAPT with aspirin and clopidogrel after coronary artery stenting can reduce the rates of in-stent restenosis without significantly affecting bleeding risk [191–193], however benefits with regards to hard clinical outcomes have not been shown.

For example, the CREST, CILON-T and DECLARE-LONG II trials each randomized patients after PCI to cilostazol plus traditional DAPT versus DAPT alone, and despite significant reductions in late lumen loss and greater reductions in platelet reactivity as measured in PRU, the addition of cilostazol to traditional DAPT did not show any benefit with regards to cardiovascular adverse events including death, MI, ischemic stroke, target lesion revascularization, or ST [194–196].

## Protease-Activated Receptor Inhibitors

Vorapaxar, a new platelet inhibitor, works as an oral competitive protease-activated receptor-1 (PAR-1) antagonist by selectively inhibiting thrombin-mediated activation of PAR-1 on platelet surfaces. It was recently evaluated as an adjunct to standard DAPT in the TRACER trial, which enrolled 12,944 patients with NSTE-ACS, randomizing them to treatment with vorapaxar (40 mg loading dose followed by 2.5 mg daily thereafter) plus aspirin and clopidogrel versus standard DAPT [197]. The trial was terminated early after a safety review found significantly higher rates of moderate to severe bleeding (7.2% vs. 5.2%, p<0.001), including intracranial hemorrhages (1.1% vs. 0.2%, p<0.001), without any counterbalancing benefit with regards to the primary composite endpoint of cardiac death, MI, stroke, recurrent ischemia with rehospitalization, or urgent coronary revascularization (18.5% vs. 19.9%, p=0.07). There was also no difference in the secondary end point of ST (1.7% vs. 1.5%, p=0.54).

## Factor Xa Inhibitors

Rivaroxaban is an oral anticoagulant that directly inhibits factor Xa. It is currently approved for use in the United States for the prevention of deep venous thrombosis and pulmonary embolism in patients who have undergone hip and knee replacement surgeries, as well as for the prevention of strokes in nonvalvular atrial fibrillation. ATLAS ACS 2 TIMI 51 was a large trial that enrolled 15,526 patients to evaluate the effect of rivaroxaban on cardiovascular outcomes after a recent ACS [198]. The patients were randomized to twice daily doses of either 2.5 mg or 5 mg of rivaroxaban versus placebo for a mean of 13 months and up to 31 months. Rivaroxaban at both doses significantly reduced the primary composite endpoint of cardiac death, MI or stroke, while the twice daily 2.5 mg dose of rivaroxaban decreased both cardiovascular death as well as death from any cause. In addition, rivaroxaban reduced the risk of ST as compared with placebo (2.3% vs. 2.9%, HR 0.69, 95% CI, 0.51 to 0.93, p=0.02). Despite these promising results, the drug was ultimately not approved by the FDA for the indication of ACS due to significantly higher rates of major bleeding not related to CABG (2.1% vs. 0.6%, p<0.001) and intracranial hemorrhage (0.6% vs. 0.2%, p=0.009). Additional concerns were raised about issues relating to data quality, including a high rate of incomplete patient follow-up (average rate of 12%) with close to 1,300 patients discontinuing the trial early [199].

Apixaban is another direct Xa inhibitor, which is currently approved for use in Europe to prevent venous thromboembolism after hip and knee surgery. Its use to prevent stroke in patients with atrial fibrillation has been studied and is currently undergoing review for approval by the FDA. Apixaban has also been studied as an adjunct to antiplatelet therapy in patients with ACS in the APPRAISE-2 trial, however the trial was terminated early after recruitment of 7,392 patients due to an increase in major bleeding events without any meaningful counterbalance in the reduction of recurrent ischemic events [200].

## Conflict of Interest Disclosures

Dr. Feldman is a consultant for Maquet Cardiovascular, Gilead Sciences and is a member of speaker bureau for Eli Lilly, Daiichi-Sankyo, Abbott Vascular, and The Medicines Company.

Other authors – no relevant conflicts.

## Conclusion

There has been recent strong evidence suggesting that newer generation antiplatelet agents such as prasugrel and ticagrelor may improve outcomes and reduce ischemic events when compared to clopidogrel in patients undergoing PCI. It is clear though, that certain subgroups of patients may still fare worse due to an increased risk for bleeding. Future studies will be useful to further define the long-term outcomes and safety profiles of these drugs and may provide clarity as to which anti-platelet agent to choose for specific patient groups and clinical scenarios. Important considerations in optimizing the benefit-to-risk profile of antiplatelet therapy are finding the right doses as well as limiting the duration of maintenance therapy. Ongoing research into the application of genetic and platelet function testing will help guide the practice of personalizing therapy to patients based on individual characteristics of drug responsiveness including predisposition to adverse effects and/or specific drug-drug interactions. Whom to test and what level of platelet inhibition to target are questions that require further elucidation. As newer generation coronary stents are developed, improved stent design and more effectively eluted drugs may help to shorten the duration of DAPT necessary, thereby decreasing the chance for bleeding. The search for newer and more potent anti-thrombotic drugs that minimize bleeding risk will remain a cornerstone of pharmacologic and clinical research, with ongoing studies examining new generations of $P2Y_{12}$ inhibitors, PAR-1 antagonists, and a variety of novel anticoagulants targeting different sites along the coagulation cascade.

# References

[1]    van Werkum JW, Heestermans AA, Zomer AC, Kelder JC, Suttorp M-J, Rensing BJ, et al. Predictors of coronary stent thrombosis: the Dutch Stent Thrombosis Registry. *J. Am. Coll. Cardiol.,* 2009 Apr 21;53(16):1399–409.

[2]    Armstrong EJ, Feldman DN, Wang TY, Kaltenbach LA, Yeo K-K, Wong SC, et al. Clinical presentation, management, and outcomes of angiographically documented early, late, and very late stent thrombosis. *JACC Cardiovasc. Interv.,* 2012 Feb;5(2):131–40.

[3]    Kolandaivelu K, Swaminathan R, Gibson WJ, Kolachalama VB, Nguyen-Ehrenreich K-L, Giddings VL, et al. Stent thrombogenicity early in high-risk interventional settings is driven by stent design and deployment and protected by polymer-drug coatings. *Circulation,* 2011 Apr 5;123(13):1400–9.

[4]    Lagerqvist B, James SK, Stenestrand U, Lindbäck J, Nilsson T, Wallentin L. Long-term outcomes with drug-eluting stents versus bare-metal stents in Sweden. *N. Engl. J. Med.,* 2007 Mar 8;356(10):1009–19.

[5]    Moreno R, Fernández C, Hernández R, Alfonso F, Angiolillo DJ, Sabaté M, et al. Drug-eluting stent thrombosis: results from a pooled analysis including 10 randomized studies. *J. Am. Coll. Cardiol.,* 2005 Mar 15;45(6):954–9.

[6]   Roiron C, Sanchez P, Bouzamondo A, Lechat P, Montalescot G. Drug eluting stents: an updated meta-analysis of randomised controlled trials. *Heart,* 2006 May;92(5):641–9.

[7]   Weisz G, Leon MB, Holmes DR, Kereiakes DJ, Popma JJ, Teirstein PS, et al. Five-year follow-up after sirolimus-eluting stent implantation results of the SIRIUS (Sirolimus-Eluting Stent in De-Novo Native Coronary Lesions) Trial. *J. Am. Coll. Cardiol.,* 2009 Apr 28;53(17): 1488–97.

[8]   Cairns JA, Gent M, Singer J, Finnie KJ, Froggatt GM, Holder DA, et al. Aspirin, sulfinpyrazone, or both in unstable angina. Results of a Canadian multicenter trial. *N. Engl. J. Med.,* 1985 Nov 28;313(22): 1369–75.

[9]   Lewis HD, Davis JW, Archibald DG, Steinke WE, Smitherman TC, Doherty JE, et al. Protective effects of aspirin against acute myocardial infarction and death in men with unstable angina. Results of a Veterans Administration Cooperative Study. *N. Engl. J. Med.,* 1983 Aug 18;309 (7):396–403.

[10]  Théroux P, Ouimet H, McCans J, Latour JG, Joly P, Lévy G, et al. Aspirin, heparin, or both to treat acute unstable angina. *N. Engl. J. Med.,* 1988 Oct 27;319(17):1105–11.

[11]  Randomised trial of intravenous streptokinase, oral aspirin, both, or neither among 17,187 cases of suspected acute myocardial infarction: ISIS-2. ISIS-2 (Second International Study of Infarct Survival) Collaborative Group. *Lancet,* 1988 Aug 13;2(8607):349–60.

[12]  Risk of myocardial infarction and death during treatment with low dose aspirin and intravenous heparin in men with unstable coronary artery disease. The RISC Group. *Lancet,* 1990 Oct 6;336(8719):827–30.

[13]  Schwartz L, Bourassa MG, Lespérance J, Aldridge HE, Kazim F, Salvatori VA, et al. Aspirin and dipyridamole in the prevention of restenosis after percutaneous transluminal coronary angioplasty. *N. Engl. J. Med.,* 1988 Jun 30;318(26):1714–9.

[14]  Lembo NJ, Black AJ, Roubin GS, Wilentz JR, Mufson LH, Douglas JS, et al. Effect of pretreatment with aspirin versus aspirin plus dipyridamole on frequency and type of acute complications of percutaneous transluminal coronary angioplasty. *Am. J. Cardiol.,* 1990 Feb 15;65(7):422–6.

[15]  Mufson, L, Black, A, Roubin, G et al. A randomized trial of aspirin in PTCA: effect of high dose versus low dose aspirin on major

complications and restenosis (abstract). *J. Am. Coll. Cardiol.*, 1988;11 (236A).

[16]  Levine GN, Bates ER, Blankenship JC, Bailey SR, Bittl JA, Cercek B, et al. 2011 ACCF/AHA/SCAI Guideline for Percutaneous Coronary Intervention. A report of the American College of Cardiology Foundation/American Heart Association Task Force on Practice Guidelines and the Society for Cardiovascular Angiography and Interventions. *J. Am. Coll. Cardiol.*, 2011 Dec 6;58(24):e44–122.

[17]  Balsano F, Rizzon P, Violi F, Scrutinio D, Cimminiello C, Aguglia F, et al. Antiplatelet treatment with ticlopidine in unstable angina. A controlled multicenter clinical trial. The Studio della Ticlopidina nell'Angina Instabile Group. *Circulation,* 1990 Jul;82(1):17–26.

[18]  Bertrand ME, Legrand V, Boland J, Fleck E, Bonnier J, Emmanuelson H, et al. Randomized multicenter comparison of conventional anticoagulation versus antiplatelet therapy in unplanned and elective coronary stenting. The full anticoagulation versus aspirin and ticlopidine (fantastic) study. *Circulation,* 1998 Oct 20;98(16):1597–603.

[19]  Leon MB, Baim DS, Popma JJ, Gordon PC, Cutlip DE, Ho KK, et al. A clinical trial comparing three antithrombotic-drug regimens after coronary-artery stenting. Stent Anticoagulation Restenosis Study Investigators. *N. Engl. J. Med.,* 1998 Dec 3;339(23):1665–71.

[20]  Schömig A, Neumann FJ, Kastrati A, Schühlen H, Blasini R, Hadamitzky M, et al. A randomized comparison of antiplatelet and anticoagulant therapy after the placement of coronary-artery stents. *N. Engl. J. Med.,* 1996 Apr 25;334(17):1084–9.

[21]  Urban P, Macaya C, Rupprecht HJ, Kiemeneij F, Emanuelsson H, Fontanelli A, et al. Randomized evaluation of anticoagulation versus antiplatelet therapy after coronary stent implantation in high-risk patients: the multicenter aspirin and ticlopidine trial after intracoronary stenting (MATTIS). *Circulation,* 1998 Nov 17;98(20):2126–32.

[22]  Bennett CL, Davidson CJ, Raisch DW, Weinberg PD, Bennett RH, Feldman MD. Thrombotic thrombocytopenic purpura associated with ticlopidine in the setting of coronary artery stents and stroke prevention. *Arch. Intern. Med.,* 1999 Nov 22;159(21):2524–8.

[23]  Steinhubl SR, Tan WA, Foody JM, Topol EJ. Incidence and clinical course of thrombotic thrombocytopenic purpura due to ticlopidine following coronary stenting. EPISTENT Investigators. Evaluation of Platelet IIb/IIIa Inhibitor for Stenting. *JAMA,* 1999 Mar 3;281(9): 806–10.

[24] A randomised, blinded, trial of clopidogrel versus aspirin in patients at risk of ischaemic events (CAPRIE). CAPRIE Steering Committee. *Lancet*, 1996 Nov 16;348(9038):1329–39.

[25] Bertrand ME, Rupprecht HJ, Urban P, Gershlick AH. Double-blind study of the safety of clopidogrel with and without a loading dose in combination with aspirin compared with ticlopidine in combination with aspirin after coronary stenting : the clopidogrel aspirin stent international cooperative study (CLAS. *Circulation*, 2000 Aug 8;102(6):624–9.

[26] Bhatt DL, Bertrand ME, Berger PB, L'Allier PL, Moussa I, Moses JW, et al. Meta-analysis of randomized and registry comparisons of ticlopidine with clopidogrel after stenting. *J. Am. Coll. Cardiol.*, 2002 Jan 2;39(1):9–14.

[27] Yusuf S, Zhao F, Mehta SR, Chrolavicius S, Tognoni G, Fox KK. Effects of clopidogrel in addition to aspirin in patients with acute coronary syndromes without ST-segment elevation. *N. Engl. J. Med.*, 2001 Aug 16;345(7):494–502.

[28] Mehta SR, Yusuf S, Peters RJ, Bertrand ME, Lewis BS, Natarajan MK, et al. Effects of pretreatment with clopidogrel and aspirin followed by long-term therapy in patients undergoing percutaneous coronary intervention: the PCI-CURE study. *Lancet*, 2001 Aug 18;358(9281): 527–33.

[29] Yusuf S, Mehta SR, Zhao F, Gersh BJ, Commerford PJ, Blumenthal M, et al. Early and late effects of clopidogrel in patients with acute coronary syndromes. *Circulation*, 2003 Feb 25;107(7):966–72.

[30] Steinhubl SR, Berger PB, Mann JT, Fry ETA, DeLago A, Wilmer C, et al. Early and sustained dual oral antiplatelet therapy following percutaneous coronary intervention: a randomized controlled trial. *JAMA*, 2002 Nov 20;288(19):2411–20.

[31] Sabatine MS, Cannon CP, Gibson CM, López-Sendón JL, Montalescot G, Theroux P, et al. Addition of clopidogrel to aspirin and fibrinolytic therapy for myocardial infarction with ST-segment elevation. *N. Engl. J. Med.*, 2005 Mar 24;352(12):1179–89.

[32] Chen ZM, Jiang LX, Chen YP, Xie JX, Pan HC, Peto R, et al. Addition of clopidogrel to aspirin in 45,852 patients with acute myocardial infarction: randomised placebo-controlled trial. *Lancet*, 2005 Nov 5;366(9497):1607–21.

[33] Sabatine MS, Cannon CP, Gibson CM, López-Sendón JL, Montalescot G, Theroux P, et al. Effect of clopidogrel pretreatment before

percutaneous coronary intervention in patients with ST-elevation myocardial infarction treated with fibrinolytics: the PCI-CLARITY study. *JAMA,* 2005 Sep 14;294(10):1224–32.

[34]  Steinhubl SR, Berger PB, Brennan DM, Topol EJ. Optimal timing for the initiation of pre-treatment with 300 mg clopidogrel before percutaneous coronary intervention. *J. Am. Coll. Cardiol.,* 2006 Mar 7;47(5):939–43.

[35]  Hochholzer W, Trenk D, Frundi D, Blanke P, Fischer B, Andris K, et al. Time dependence of platelet inhibition after a 600-mg loading dose of clopidogrel in a large, unselected cohort of candidates for percutaneous coronary intervention. *Circulation,* 2005 May 24;111(20):2560–4.

[36]  Angiolillo DJ, Fernández-Ortiz A, Bernardo E, Ramírez C, Sabaté M, Bañuelos C, et al. High clopidogrel loading dose during coronary stenting: effects on drug response and interindividual variability. *Eur. Heart J.,* 2004 Nov;25(21):1903–10.

[37]  Patti G, Colonna G, Pasceri V, Pepe LL, Montinaro A, Di Sciascio G. Randomized trial of high loading dose of clopidogrel for reduction of periprocedural myocardial infarction in patients undergoing coronary intervention: results from the ARMYDA-2 (Antiplatelet therapy for Reduction of MYocardial Damage during Angioplasty). *Circulation,* 2005 Apr 26;111(16):2099–106.

[38]  Dangas G, Mehran R, Guagliumi G, Caixeta A, Witzenbichler B, Aoki J, et al. Role of clopidogrel loading dose in patients with ST-segment elevation myocardial infarction undergoing primary angioplasty: results from the HORIZONS-AMI (harmonizing outcomes with revascularization and stents in acute myocardial infarction) trial. *J. Am. Coll. Cardiol.,* 2009 Oct 6;54(15):1438–46.

[39]  Mehta SR, Tanguay J-F, Eikelboom JW, Jolly SS, Joyner CD, Granger CB, et al. Double-dose versus standard-dose clopidogrel and high-dose versus low-dose aspirin in individuals undergoing percutaneous coronary intervention for acute coronary syndromes (CURRENT-OASIS 7): a randomised factorial trial. *Lancet,* 2010 Oct 9;376(9748):1233–43.

[40]  Mehta SR, Bassand J-P, Chrolavicius S, Diaz R, Eikelboom JW, Fox KAA, et al. Dose comparisons of clopidogrel and aspirin in acute coronary syndromes. *N. Engl. J. Med.,* 2010 Sep 2;363(10):930–42.

[41]  von Beckerath N, Taubert D, Pogatsa-Murray G, Schömig E, Kastrati A, Schömig A. Absorption, metabolization, and antiplatelet effects of 300-, 600-, and 900-mg loading doses of clopidogrel: results of the ISAR-CHOICE (Intracoronary Stenting and Antithrombotic Regimen: Choose

Between 3 High Oral Doses for Immediate Clopidogrel Effect). *Circulation,* 2005 Nov 8;112(19):2946–50.

[42]   Montalescot G, Sideris G, Meuleman C, Bal-dit-Sollier C, Lellouche N, Steg PG, et al. A randomized comparison of high clopidogrel loading doses in patients with non-ST-segment elevation acute coronary syndromes: the ALBION (Assessment of the Best Loading Dose of Clopidogrel to Blunt Platelet Activation, Inflammation and Ongoing Necrosis) t. *J. Am. Coll. Cardiol.,* 2006 Sep 5;48(5):931–8.

[43]   L'Allier PL, Ducrocq G, Pranno N, Noble S, Ibrahim R, Grégoire JC, et al. Clopidogrel 600-mg double loading dose achieves stronger platelet inhibition than conventional regimens: results from the PREPAIR randomized study. *J. Am. Coll. Cardiol.,* 2008 Mar 18;51(11):1066–72.

[44]   Kandzari DE, Berger PB, Kastrati A, Steinhubl SR, Mehilli J, Dotzer F, et al. Influence of treatment duration with a 600-mg dose of clopidogrel before percutaneous coronary revascularization. *J. Am. Coll. Cardiol.,* 2004 Dec 7;44(11):2133–6.

[45]   Widimsky P, Motovská Z, Simek S, Kala P, Pudil R, Holm F, et al. Clopidogrel pre-treatment in stable angina: for all patients > 6 h before elective coronary angiography or only for angiographically selected patients a few minutes before PCI? A randomized multicentre trial PRAGUE-8. *Eur. Heart J.,* 2008 Jun;29(12):1495–503.

[46]   Di Sciascio G, Patti G, Pasceri V, Gatto L, Colonna G, Montinaro A. Effectiveness of in-laboratory high-dose clopidogrel loading versus routine pre-load in patients undergoing percutaneous coronary intervention: results of the ARMYDA-5 PRELOAD (Antiplatelet therapy for Reduction of MYocardial Damage during Angioplasty) ra. *J. Am. Coll Cardiol.,* 2010 Aug 10;56(7):550–7.

[47]   Collet J-P, Silvain J, Landivier A, Tanguy M-L, Cayla G, Bellemain A, et al. Dose effect of clopidogrel reloading in patients already on 75-mg maintenance dose: the Reload with Clopidogrel Before Coronary Angioplasty in Subjects Treated Long Term with Dual Antiplatelet Therapy (RELOAD) study. *Circulation,* 2008 Sep 16;118(12):1225–33.

[48]   Di Sciascio G, Patti G, Pasceri V, Colonna G, Mangiacapra F, Montinaro A. Clopidogrel reloading in patients undergoing percutaneous coronary intervention on chronic clopidogrel therapy: results of the ARMYDA-4 RELOAD (Antiplatelet therapy for Reduction of MYocardial Damage during Angioplasty) randomized trial. *Eur. Heart J., 2010* Jun;31(11):1337–43.

[49]   Brandt JT, Payne CD, Wiviott SD, Weerakkody G, Farid NA, Small DS, et al. A comparison of prasugrel and clopidogrel loading doses on platelet function: magnitude of platelet inhibition is related to active metabolite formation. *Am. Heart J.,* 2007 Jan;153(1):66.e9–16.

[50]   Jernberg T, Payne CD, Winters KJ, Darstein C, Brandt JT, Jakubowski JA, et al. Prasugrel achieves greater inhibition of platelet aggregation and a lower rate of non-responders compared with clopidogrel in aspirin-treated patients with stable coronary artery disease. *Eur. Heart J.,* 2006 May;27(10):1166–73.

[51]   Wiviott SD, Antman EM, Winters KJ, Weerakkody G, Murphy SA, Behounek BD, et al. Randomized comparison of prasugrel (CS-747, LY640315), a novel thienopyridine P2Y12 antagonist, with clopidogrel in percutaneous coronary intervention: results of the Joint Utilization of Medications to Block Platelets Optimally (JUMBO)-TIMI 26 trial. *Circulation,* 2005 Jun 28;111(25):3366–73.

[52]   Wiviott SD, Trenk D, Frelinger AL, O'Donoghue M, Neumann F-J, Michelson AD, et al. Prasugrel compared with high loading- and maintenance-dose clopidogrel in patients with planned percutaneous coronary intervention: the Prasugrel in Comparison to Clopidogrel for Inhibition of Platelet Activation and Aggregation-Thrombolysis in Myocardial. *Circulation,* 2007 Dec 18;116(25):2923–32.

[53]   Wiviott SD, Braunwald E, McCabe CH, Montalescot G, Ruzyllo W, Gottlieb S, et al. Prasugrel versus clopidogrel in patients with acute coronary syndromes. *N. Engl. J. Med.,* 2007 Nov 15;357(20):2001–15.

[54]   Wiviott SD, Braunwald E, McCabe CH, Horvath I, Keltai M, Herrman J-PR, et al. Intensive oral antiplatelet therapy for reduction of ischaemic events including stent thrombosis in patients with acute coronary syndromes treated with percutaneous coronary intervention and stenting in the TRITON-TIMI 38 trial: a subanalysis of a randomi. *Lancet,* 2008 Apr 19;371(9621):1353–63.

[55]   O'Donoghue M, Antman EM, Braunwald E, Murphy SA, Steg PG, Finkelstein A, et al. The efficacy and safety of prasugrel with and without a glycoprotein IIb/IIIa inhibitor in patients with acute coronary syndromes undergoing percutaneous intervention: a TRITON-TIMI 38 (Trial to Assess Improvement in Therapeutic Outcomes by Optimizing Pla. *J. Am. Coll. Cardiol.,* 2009 Aug 18;54(8):678–85.

[56]   Angiolillo DJ, Capranzano P. Pharmacology of emerging novel platelet inhibitors. *Am. Heart J.,* 2008 Aug;156(2 Suppl):S10–5.

[57] Gurbel PA, Bliden KP, Butler K, Tantry US, Gesheff T, Wei C, et al. Randomized double-blind assessment of the ONSET and OFFSET of the antiplatelet effects of ticagrelor versus clopidogrel in patients with stable coronary artery disease: the ONSET/OFFSET study. *Circulation,* 2009 Dec 22;120(25):2577–85.

[58] Alexopoulos D, Galati A, Xanthopoulou I, Mavronasiou E, Kassimis G, Theodoropoulos KC, et al. Ticagrelor versus prasugrel in acute coronary syndrome patients with high on-clopidogrel platelet reactivity following percutaneous coronary intervention: a pharmacodynamic study. *J. Am. Coll. Cardiol.,* 2012 Jul 17;60(3):193–9.

[59] Wallentin L, Becker RC, Budaj A, Cannon CP, Emanuelsson H, Held C, et al. Ticagrelor versus clopidogrel in patients with acute coronary syndromes. *N. Engl. J. Med.,* 2009 Sep 10;361(11):1045–57.

[60] James S, Budaj A, Aylward P, Buck KK, Cannon CP, Cornel JH, et al. Ticagrelor versus clopidogrel in acute coronary syndromes in relation to renal function: results from the Platelet Inhibition and Patient Outcomes (PLATO) trial. *Circulation,* 2010 Sep 14;122(11):1056–67.

[61] Mahaffey KW, Wojdyla DM, Carroll K, Becker RC, Storey RF, Angiolillo DJ, et al. Ticagrelor compared with clopidogrel by geographic region in the Platelet Inhibition and Patient Outcomes (PLATO) trial. *Circulation,* 2011 Aug 2;124(5):544–54.

[62] Kushner FG, Hand M, Smith SC, King SB, Anderson JL, Antman EM, et al. 2009 Focused Updates: ACC/AHA Guidelines for the Management of Patients With ST-Elevation Myocardial Infarction (updating the 2004 Guideline and 2007 Focused Update) and ACC/AHA/SCAI Guidelines on Percutaneous Coronary Intervention (updating the 2005 Guid. *J. Am. Coll. Cardiol.,* 2009 Dec 1;120(22):2205–41.

[63] Jneid H, Anderson JL, Wright RS, Adams CD, Bridges CR, Casey DE, et al. 2012 ACCF/AHA Focused Update of the Guideline for the Management of Patients With Unstable Angina/Non-ST-Elevation Myocardial Infarction (Updating the 2007 Guideline and Replacing the 2011 Focused Update): A Report of the American College of Cardiology Fo. *J. Am. Coll. Cardiol.,* 2012 Jul 16;60(7):645–81.

[64] Järemo P, Lindahl TL, Fransson SG, Richter A. Individual variations of platelet inhibition after loading doses of clopidogrel. *J. Intern. Med.,* 2002 Sep;252(3):233–8.

[65] Gurbel PA, Becker RC, Mann KG, Steinhubl SR, Michelson AD. Platelet function monitoring in patients with coronary artery disease. *J. Am. Coll. Cardiol.,* 2007 Nov 6;50(19):1822–34.

[66]  von Beckerath N, Pogatsa-Murray G, Wieczorek A, Sibbing D, Schömig A, Kastrati A. Correlation of a new point-of-care test with conventional optical aggregometry for the assessment of clopidogrel responsiveness. *Thromb Haemost.*, 2006 May;95(5):910–1.

[67]  Godino C, Mendolicchio L, Figini F, Latib A, Sharp AS, Cosgrave J, et al. Comparison of VerifyNow-P2Y12 test and Flow Cytometry for monitoring individual platelet response to clopidogrel. What is the cut-off value for identifying patients who are low responders to clopidogrel therapy? *Thromb J.*, 2009 Jan;7:4.

[68]  Sibbing D, Morath T, Braun S, Stegherr J, Mehilli J, Vogt W, et al. Clopidogrel response status assessed with Multiplate point-of-care analysis and the incidence and timing of stent thrombosis over six months following coronary stenting. *Thromb Haemost.*, 2010 Jan;103(1):151–9.

[69]  Price MJ, Berger PB, Teirstein PS, Tanguay J-F, Angiolillo DJ, Spriggs D, et al. Standard- vs high-dose clopidogrel based on platelet function testing after percutaneous coronary intervention: the GRAVITAS randomized trial. *JAMA,* 2011 Mar 16;305(11):1097–105.

[70]  Price MJ, Angiolillo DJ, Teirstein PS, Lillie E, Manoukian SV, Berger PB, et al. Platelet reactivity and cardiovascular outcomes after percutaneous coronary intervention: a time-dependent analysis of the Gauging Responsiveness with a VerifyNow P2Y12 assay: Impact on Thrombosis and Safety (GRAVITAS) trial. *Circulation,* 2011 Sep 6;124(10):1132–7.

[71]  Trenk D, Stone GW, Gawaz M, Kastrati A, Angiolillo DJ, Müller U, et al. A Randomized Trial of Prasugrel Versus Clopidogrel in Patients With High Platelet Reactivity on Clopidogrel After Elective Percutaneous Coronary Intervention With Implantation of Drug-Eluting Stents: Results of the TRIGGER-PCI (Testing Platelet Reactivity. *J. Am. Coll. Cardiol.,* 2012 Jun 12;59(24):2159–64.

[72]  Price MJ, Murray SS, Angiolillo DJ, Lillie E, Smith EN, Tisch RL, et al. Influence of genetic polymorphisms on the effect of high- and standard-dose clopidogrel after percutaneous coronary intervention: the GIFT (Genotype Information and Functional Testing) study. *J. Am. Coll. Cardiol.,* 2012 May 29;59(22):1928–37.

[73]  Mega JL, Close SL, Wiviott SD, Shen L, Hockett RD, Brandt JT, et al. Cytochrome p-450 polymorphisms and response to clopidogrel. *N. Engl. J. Med.,* 2009 Jan 22;360(4):354–62.

[74] Holmes MV, Perel P, Shah T, Hingorani AD, Casas JP. CYP2C19 genotype, clopidogrel metabolism, platelet function, and cardiovascular events: a systematic review and meta-analysis. *JAMA,* 2011 Dec 28;306(24):2704–14.

[75] Oler A, Whooley MA, Oler J, Grady D. Adding heparin to aspirin reduces the incidence of myocardial infarction and death in patients with unstable angina. A meta-analysis. *JAMA,* 1996 Sep 11;276(10):811–5.

[76] Cohen M, Adams PC, Parry G, Xiong J, Chamberlain D, Wieczorek I, et al. Combination antithrombotic therapy in unstable rest angina and non-Q-wave infarction in nonprior aspirin users. Primary end points analysis from the ATACS trial. Antithrombotic Therapy in Acute Coronary Syndromes Research Group. *Circulation,* 1994 Jan;89(1):81–8.

[77] Eikelboom JW, Anand SS, Malmberg K, Weitz JI, Ginsberg JS, Yusuf S. Unfractionated heparin and low-molecular-weight heparin in acute coronary syndrome without ST elevation: a meta-analysis. *Lancet.* 2000 Jun 3;355(9219):1936–42.

[78] Popma JJ, Weitz J, Bittl JA, Ohman EM, Kuntz RE, Lansky AJ, et al. Antithrombotic therapy in patients undergoing coronary angioplasty. *Chest,* 1998 Nov;114(5 Suppl):728S–741S.

[79] de Bono DP, Simoons ML, Tijssen J, Arnold AE, Betriu A, Burgersdijk C, et al. Effect of early intravenous heparin on coronary patency, infarct size, and bleeding complications after alteplase thrombolysis: results of a randomised double blind European Cooperative Study Group trial. *Br. Heart J.,* 1992 Feb;67(2):122–8.

[80] Arnout J, Simoons M, de Bono D, Rapold HJ, Collen D, Verstraete M. Correlation between level of heparinization and patency of the infarct-related coronary artery after treatment of acute myocardial infarction with alteplase (rt-PA). *J. Am. Coll. Cardiol.,* 1992 Sep;20(3):513–9.

[81] Eikelboom JW, Quinlan DJ, Mehta SR, Turpie AG, Menown IB, Yusuf S. Unfractionated and low-molecular-weight heparin as adjuncts to thrombolysis in aspirin-treated patients with ST-elevation acute myocardial infarction: a meta-analysis of the randomized trials. *Circulation,* 2005 Dec 20;112(25):3855–67.

[82] An international randomized trial comparing four thrombolytic strategies for acute myocardial infarction. The GUSTO investigators. *N. Engl. J. Med.,* 1993 Sep 2;329(10):673–82.

[83] Smith SC, Feldman TE, Hirshfeld JW, Jacobs AK, Kern MJ, King SB, et al. ACC/AHA/SCAI 2005 guideline update for percutaneous coronary intervention: a report of the American College of Cardiology/American

Heart Association Task Force on Practice Guidelines (ACC/AHA/SCAI Writing Committee to Update 2001 Guidelines for Percutaneo. *Circulation,* 2006 Feb 21;113(7):e166–286.

[84]  Silber S, Albertsson P, Avilés FF, Camici PG, Colombo A, Hamm C, et al. Guidelines for percutaneous coronary interventions. The Task Force for Percutaneous Coronary Interventions of the European Society of Cardiology. *Eur. Heart J.,* 2005 Apr;26(8):804–47.

[85]  Low-molecular-weight heparin during instability in coronary artery disease, Fragmin during Instability in Coronary Artery Disease (FRISC) study group. *Lancet,* 1996 Mar 2;347(9001):561–8.

[86]  Klein W, Buchwald A, Hillis SE, Monrad S, Sanz G, Turpie AG, et al. Comparison of low-molecular-weight heparin with unfractionated heparin acutely and with placebo for 6 weeks in the management of unstable coronary artery disease. Fragmin in unstable coronary artery disease study (FRIC). *Circulation,* 1997 Jul 1;96(1):61–8.

[87]  Comparison of two treatment durations (6 days and 14 days) of a low molecular weight heparin with a 6-day treatment of unfractionated heparin in the initial management of unstable angina or non-Q wave myocardial infarction: FRAX.I.S. (FRAxiparine in Ischa. *Eur. Heart J.,* 1999 Nov;20(21):1553–62.

[88]  Antman EM, Cohen M, Radley D, McCabe C, Rush J, Premmereur J, et al. Assessment of the treatment effect of enoxaparin for unstable angina/non-Q-wave myocardial infarction. TIMI 11B-ESSENCE meta-analysis. *Circulation,* 1999 Oct 12;100(15):1602–8.

[89]  Murphy SA, Gibson CM, Morrow DA, Van de Werf F, Menown IB, Goodman SG, et al. Efficacy and safety of the low-molecular weight heparin enoxaparin compared with unfractionated heparin across the acute coronary syndrome spectrum: a meta-analysis. *Eur. Heart J.,* 2007 Sep;28(17):2077–86.

[90]  Antman EM, McCabe CH, Gurfinkel EP, Turpie AG, Bernink PJ, Salein D, et al. Enoxaparin prevents death and cardiac ischemic events in unstable angina/non-Q-wave myocardial infarction. Results of the thrombolysis in myocardial infarction (TIMI) 11B trial. *Circulation,* 1999 Oct 12;100(15):1593–601.

[91]  Cohen M, Demers C, Gurfinkel EP, Turpie AG, Fromell GJ, Goodman S, et al. A comparison of low-molecular-weight heparin with unfractionated heparin for unstable coronary artery disease. Efficacy and Safety of Subcutaneous Enoxaparin in Non-Q-Wave Coronary Events Study Group. *N. Engl. J. Med.,* 1997 Aug 14;337(7):447–52.

[92]  Ferguson JJ, Califf RM, Antman EM, Cohen M, Grines CL, Goodman S, et al. Enoxaparin vs unfractionated heparin in high-risk patients with non-ST-segment elevation acute coronary syndromes managed with an intended early invasive strategy: primary results of the SYNERGY randomized trial. *JAMA*, 2004 Jul 7;292(1):45–54.

[93]  Montalescot G, White HD, Gallo R, Cohen M, Steg PG, Aylward PEG, et al. Enoxaparin versus unfractionated heparin in elective percutaneous coronary intervention. *N. Engl. J. Med.*, 2006 Sep 7;355(10):1006–17.

[94]  Mehta SR, Steg PG, Granger CB, Bassand J-P, Faxon DP, Weitz JI, et al. Randomized, blinded trial comparing fondaparinux with unfractionated heparin in patients undergoing contemporary percutaneous coronary intervention: Arixtra Study in Percutaneous Coronary Intervention: a Randomized Evaluation (ASPIRE) *Pilot. Trial. Circulation*, 2005 Mar 22;111(11):1390–7.

[95]  Yusuf S, Mehta SR, Chrolavicius S, Afzal R, Pogue J, Granger CB, et al. Effects of fondaparinux on mortality and reinfarction in patients with acute ST-segment elevation myocardial infarction: the OASIS-6 randomized trial. *JAMA*, 2006 Apr 5;295(13):1519–30.

[96]  King SB, Smith SC, Hirshfeld JW, Jacobs AK, Morrison DA, Williams DO, et al. 2007 Focused Update of the ACC/AHA/SCAI 2005 Guideline Update for Percutaneous Coronary Intervention: a report of the American College of Cardiology/American Heart Association Task Force on Practice Guidelines: 2007 Writing Group to Review New Evidence an. *Circulation*, 2008 Jan 15;117(2):261–95.

[97]  Weitz JI, Hudoba M, Massel D, Maraganore J, Hirsh J. Clot-bound thrombin is protected from inhibition by heparin-antithrombin III but is susceptible to inactivation by antithrombin III-independent inhibitors. *J. Clin. Invest.*, 1990 Aug;86(2):385–91.

[98]  Antman EM. Hirudin in acute myocardial infarction. Thrombolysis and Thrombin Inhibition in Myocardial Infarction (TIMI) 9B trial. *Circulation*, 1996 Sep 1;94(5):911–21.

[99]  A comparison of recombinant hirudin with heparin for the treatment of acute coronary syndromes. The Global Use of Strategies to Open Occluded Coronary Arteries (GUSTO) IIb investigators. *N. Engl. J. Med.*, 1996 Sep 12;335(11):775–82.

[100] Serruys PW, Herrman JP, Simon R, Rutsch W, Bode C, Laarman GJ, et al. A comparison of hirudin with heparin in the prevention of restenosis after coronary angioplasty. Helvetica Investigators. *N. Engl. J. Med.*, 1995 Sep 21;333(12):757–63.

[101] White HD, Aylward PE, Frey MJ, Adgey AA, Nair R, Hillis WS, et al. Randomized, double-blind comparison of hirulog versus heparin in patients receiving streptokinase and aspirin for acute myocardial infarction (HERO). Hirulog Early Reperfusion/Occlusion (HERO) Trial Investigators. *Circulation,* 1997 Oct 7;96(7):2155–61.

[102] White H. Thrombin-specific anticoagulation with bivalirudin versus heparin in patients receiving fibrinolytic therapy for acute myocardial infarction: the HERO-2 randomised trial. *Lancet,* 2001 Dec 1;358(9296):1855–63.

[103] Stone GW, Witzenbichler B, Guagliumi G, Peruga JZ, Brodie BR, Dudek D, et al. Bivalirudin during primary PCI in acute myocardial infarction. *N. Engl. J. Med.,* 2008 May 22;358(21):2218–30.

[104] Lincoff AM, Bittl JA, Harrington RA, Feit F, Kleiman NS, Jackman JD, et al. Bivalirudin and provisional glycoprotein IIb/IIIa blockade compared with heparin and planned glycoprotein IIb/IIIa blockade during percutaneous coronary intervention: REPLACE-2 randomized trial. *JAMA,* 2003 Feb 19;289(7):853–63.

[105] Kastrati A, Neumann F-J, Mehilli J, Byrne RA, Iijima R, Büttner HJ, et al. Bivalirudin versus unfractionated heparin during percutaneous coronary intervention. *N. Engl. J. Med.,* 2008 Aug 14;359(7):688–96.

[106] Stone GW, McLaurin BT, Cox DA, Bertrand ME, Lincoff AM, Moses JW, et al. Bivalirudin for patients with acute coronary syndromes. *N. Engl. J. Med.,* 2006 Nov 23;355(21):2203–16.

[107] Chew DP, Bhatt DL, Kimball W, Henry TD, Berger P, McCullough PA, et al. Bivalirudin provides increasing benefit with decreasing renal function: a meta-analysis of randomized trials. *Am. J. Cardiol.,* 2003 Oct 15;92(8):919–23.

[108] Use of a monoclonal antibody directed against the platelet glycoprotein IIb/IIIa receptor in high-risk coronary angioplasty. The EPIC Investigation. *N. Engl. J. Med.,* 1994 Apr 7;330(14):956–61.

[109] Lincoff AM, Tcheng JE, Califf RM, Kereiakes DJ, Kelly TA, Timmis GC, et al. Sustained suppression of ischemic complications of coronary intervention by platelet GP IIb/IIIa blockade with abciximab: one-year outcome in the EPILOG trial. Evaluation in PTCA to Improve Long-term Outcome with abciximab GP IIb/IIIa blockade. *Circulation,* 1999 Apr 20;99(15):1951–8.

[110] Randomised placebo-controlled trial of abciximab before and during coronary intervention in refractory unstable angina: the CAPTURE Study. *Lancet,* 1997 May 17;349(9063):1429–35.

[111] Brener SJ, Barr LA, Burchenal JE, Katz S, George BS, Jones AA, et al. Randomized, placebo-controlled trial of platelet glycoprotein IIb/IIIa blockade with primary angioplasty for acute myocardial infarction. ReoPro and Primary PTCA Organization and Randomized Trial (RAPPORT) Investigators. *Circulation,* 1998 Aug 25;98(8):734–41.

[112] Montalescot G, Barragan P, Wittenberg O, Ecollan P, Elhadad S, Villain P, et al. Platelet glycoprotein IIb/IIIa inhibition with coronary stenting for acute myocardial infarction. *N. Engl. J. Med.,* 2001 Jun 21;344(25): 1895–903.

[113] Neumann FJ, Kastrati A, Schmitt C, Blasini R, Hadamitzky M, Mehilli J, et al. Effect of glycoprotein IIb/IIIa receptor blockade with abciximab on clinical and angiographic restenosis rate after the placement of coronary stents following acute myocardial infarction. *J. Am. Coll. Cardiol.,* 2000 Mar 15;35(4):915–21.

[114] Stone GW, Grines CL, Cox DA, Garcia E, Tcheng JE, Griffin JJ, et al. Comparison of angioplasty with stenting, with or without abciximab, in acute myocardial infarction. *N. Engl. J. Med.,* 2002 Mar 28;346(13): 957–66.

[115] Antoniucci D, Rodriguez A, Hempel A, Valenti R, Migliorini A, Vigo F, et al. A randomized trial comparing primary infarct artery stenting with or without abciximab in acute myocardial infarction. *J. Am. Coll. Cardiol.,* 2003 Dec 3;42(11):1879–85.

[116] Randomised placebo-controlled and balloon-angioplasty-controlled trial to assess safety of coronary stenting with use of platelet glycoprotein-IIb/IIIa blockade. *Lancet,* 1998 Jul 11;352(9122):87–92.

[117] Kastrati A, Mehilli J, Schühlen H, Dirschinger J, Dotzer F, ten Berg JM, et al. A clinical trial of abciximab in elective percutaneous coronary intervention after pretreatment with clopidogrel. *N. Engl. J. Med.,* 2004 Jan 15;350(3):232–8.

[118] Mehilli J, Kastrati A, Schühlen H, Dibra A, Dotzer F, von Beckerath N, et al. Randomized clinical trial of abciximab in diabetic patients undergoing elective percutaneous coronary interventions after treatment with a high loading dose of clopidogrel. *Circulation,* 2004 Dec 14;110(24):3627–35.

[119] Acute platelet inhibition with abciximab does not reduce in-stent restenosis (ERASER study). The ERASER Investigators. *Circulation,* 1999 Aug 24;100(8):799–806.

[120] Bhatt DL, Lincoff AM, Califf RM, Simoons ML, Tcheng JE, Brener SJ, et al. The benefit of abciximab in percutaneous coronary

revascularization is not device-specific. *Am. J. Cardiol.*, 2000 May 1;85(9):1060–4.

[121] Cho L, Topol EJ, Balog C, Foody JM, Booth JE, Cabot C, et al. Clinical benefit of glycoprotein IIb/IIIa blockade with Abciximab is independent of gender: pooled analysis from EPIC, EPILOG and EPISTENT trials. Evaluation of 7E3 for the Prevention of Ischemic Complications. Evaluation in Percutaneous Transluminal Coro. *J. Am. Coll. Cardiol.*, 2000 Aug;36(2):381–6.

[122] Topol EJ, Lincoff AM, Kereiakes DJ, Kleiman NS, Cohen EA, Ferguson JJ, et al. Multi-year follow-up of abciximab therapy in three randomized, placebo-controlled trials of percutaneous coronary revascularization. *Am. J. Med.*, 2002 Jul;113(1):1–6.

[123] Mehilli J, Kastrati A, Schulz S, Früngel S, Nekolla SG, Moshage W, et al. Abciximab in patients with acute ST-segment-elevation myocardial infarction undergoing primary percutaneous coronary intervention after clopidogrel loading: a randomized double-blind trial. *Circulation*, 2009 Apr 14;119(14):1933–40.

[124] Effects of platelet glycoprotein IIb/IIIa blockade with tirofiban on adverse cardiac events in patients with unstable angina or acute myocardial infarction undergoing coronary angioplasty. The RESTORE Investigators. Randomized Efficacy Study of Tirofiban. *Circulation*, 1997 Sep 2;96(5):1445–53.

[125] Gibson CM, Goel M, Cohen DJ, Piana RN, Deckelbaum LI, Harris KE, et al. Six-month angiographic and clinical follow-up of patients prospectively randomized to receive either tirofiban or placebo during angioplasty in the RESTORE trial. Randomized Efficacy Study of Tirofiban for Outcomes and Restenosis. *J. Am. Coll. Cardiol.*, 1998 Jul;32 (1):28–34.

[126] Valgimigli M, Percoco G, Barbieri D, Ferrari F, Guardigli G, Parrinello G, et al. The additive value of tirofiban administered with the high-dose bolus in the prevention of ischemic complications during high-risk coronary angioplasty: the ADVANCE Trial. *J. Am. Coll. Cardiol.*, 2004 Jul 7;44(1):14–9.

[127] Lee DP, Herity NA, Hiatt BL, Fearon WF, Rezaee M, Carter AJ, et al. Adjunctive platelet glycoprotein IIb/IIIa receptor inhibition with tirofiban before primary angioplasty improves angiographic outcomes: results of the TIrofiban Given in the Emergency Room before Primary Angioplasty (TIGER-PA) pilot trial. *Circulation*, 2003 Mar 25;107(11):1497–501.

[128] van't Hof AWJ, Ernst N, de Boer M-J, de Winter R, Boersma E, Bunt T, et al. Facilitation of primary coronary angioplasty by early start of a glycoprotein 2b/3a inhibitor: results of the ongoing tirofiban in myocardial infarction evaluation (On-TIME) trial. *Eur. Heart J.,* 2004 May;25(10):837–46.

[129] van't Hof AWJ, Ten Berg J, Heestermans T, Dill T, Funck RC, van Werkum W, et al. Prehospital initiation of tirofiban in patients with ST-elevation myocardial infarction undergoing primary angioplasty (On-TIME 2): a multicentre, double-blind, randomised controlled trial. *Lancet,* 2008 Aug 16;372(9638):537–46.

[130] ten Berg JM, van 't Hof AWJ, Dill T, Heestermans T, van Werkum JW, Mosterd A, et al. Effect of early, pre-hospital initiation of high bolus dose tirofiban in patients with ST-segment elevation myocardial infarction on short- and long-term clinical outcome. *J. Am. Coll. Cardiol.,* 2010 Jun 1;55(22):2446–55.

[131] Phillips DR, Scarborough RM. Clinical pharmacology of eptifibatide. *Am. J. Cardiol.,* 1997 Aug 18;80(4A):11B–20B.

[132] Inhibition of platelet glycoprotein IIb/IIIa with eptifibatide in patients with acute coronary syndromes. The PURSUIT Trial Investigators. Platelet Glycoprotein IIb/IIIa in Unstable Angina: Receptor Suppression Using Integrilin Therapy. *N. Engl. J. Med.,* 1998 Aug 13;339(7):436–43.

[133] Kleiman NS, Lincoff AM, Flaker GC, Pieper KS, Wilcox RG, Berdan LG, et al. Early percutaneous coronary intervention, platelet inhibition with eptifibatide, and clinical outcomes in patients with acute coronary syndromes. PURSUIT Investigators. *Circulation,* 2000 Feb 22;101(7):751–7.

[134] Randomised placebo-controlled trial of effect of eptifibatide on complications of percutaneous coronary intervention: IMPACT-II. Integrilin to Minimise Platelet Aggregation and Coronary Thrombosis-II. *Lancet,* 1997 May 17;349(9063):1422–8.

[135] Novel dosing regimen of eptifibatide in planned coronary stent implantation (ESPRIT): a randomised, placebo-controlled trial. *Lancet,* 2000 Dec 16;356(9247):2037–44.

[136] Dasgupta H, Blankenship JC, Wood GC, Frey CM, Demko SL, Menapace FJ. Thrombocytopenia complicating treatment with intravenous glycoprotein IIb/IIIa receptor inhibitors: a pooled analysis. *Am. Heart J.,* 2000 Aug;140(2):206–11.

[137] Sabatine MS, Jang IK. The use of glycoprotein IIb/IIIa inhibitors in patients with coronary artery disease. *Am. J. Med.,* 2000 Aug 15;109 (3):224–37.

[138] Dangas GD, Lansky AJ, Brodie BR et al. Predictors of stent thrombosis after primary angioplasty in acute myocardial infarction. The HORIZONS-AMI Trial. p. Paper presented at: American College of Cardiology.

[139] Montalescot G, Borentain M, Payot L, Collet JP, Thomas D. Early vs late administration of glycoprotein IIb/IIIa inhibitors in primary percutaneous coronary intervention of acute ST-segment elevation myocardial infarction: a meta-analysis. *JAMA,* 2004 Jul 21;292(3):362–6.

[140] Ellis SG, Tendera M, de Belder MA, van Boven AJ, Widimsky P, Janssens L, et al. Facilitated PCI in patients with ST-elevation myocardial infarction. *N. Engl. J. Med.,* 2008 May 22;358(21):2205–17.

[141] Memon MA, Blankenship JC, Wood GC, Frey CM, Menapace FJ. Incidence of intracranial hemorrhage complicating treatment with glycoprotein IIb/IIIa receptor inhibitors: a pooled analysis of major clinical trials. *Am. J. Med.,* 2000 Aug 15;109(3):213–7.

[142] Batchelor WB, Tolleson TR, Huang Y, Larsen RL, Mantell RM, Dillard P, et al. Randomized COMparison of platelet inhibition with abciximab, tiRofiban and eptifibatide during percutaneous coronary intervention in acute coronary syndromes: the COMPARE trial. Comparison Of Measurements of Platelet aggregation with Aggrastat, Reopro, an. *Circulation,* 2002 Sep 17;106(12):1470–6.

[143] Topol EJ, Moliterno DJ, Herrmann HC, Powers ER, Grines CL, Cohen DJ, et al. Comparison of two platelet glycoprotein IIb/IIIa inhibitors, tirofiban and abciximab, for the prevention of ischemic events with percutaneous coronary revascularization. *N. Engl. J. Med.,* 2001 Jun 21;344 (25):1888–94.

[144] Moliterno DJ, Yakubov SJ, DiBattiste PM, Herrmann HC, Stone GW, Macaya C, et al. Outcomes at 6 months for the direct comparison of tirofiban and abciximab during percutaneous coronary revascularisation with stent placement: the TARGET follow-up study. *Lancet,* 2002 Aug 3;360(9330):355–60.

[145] Mukherjee D, Topol EJ, Bertrand ME, Kristensen SD, Herrmann HC, Neumann F-J, et al. Mortality at 1 year for the direct comparison of tirofiban and abciximab during percutaneous coronary revascularization:

do tirofiban and ReoPro give similar efficacy outcomes at trial 1-year follow-up. *Eur. Heart J.*, 2005 Dec;26(23):2524–8.

[146] Valgimigli M, Campo G, Percoco G, Bolognese L, Vassanelli C, Colangelo S, et al. Comparison of angioplasty with infusion of tirofiban or abciximab and with implantation of sirolimus-eluting or uncoated stents for acute myocardial infarction: the MULTISTRATEGY randomized trial. *JAMA*, 2008 Apr 16;299(15):1788–99.

[147] Midei MG, Coombs VJ, Lowry DR, Drossner MN, Prewitt KC, Wang JC, et al. Clinical outcomes comparing eptifibatide and abciximab in ST elevation acute myocardial infarction patients undergoing percutaneous coronary interventions. *Cardiology*, 2007 Jan;107(3):172–7.

[148] Effectiveness of intravenous thrombolytic treatment in acute myocardial infarction. Gruppo Italiano per lo Studio della Streptochinasi nell'Infarto Miocardico (GISSI). *Lancet*, 1986 Feb 22;1(8478):397–402.

[149] Boersma E, Maas AC, Deckers JW, Simoons ML. Early thrombolytic treatment in acute myocardial infarction: reappraisal of the golden hour. *Lancet*, 1996 Sep 21;348(9030):771–5.

[150] Franzosi MG, Santoro E, De Vita C, Geraci E, Lotto A, Maggioni AP, et al. Ten-year follow-up of the first megatrial testing thrombolytic therapy in patients with acute myocardial infarction: results of the Gruppo Italiano per lo Studio della Sopravvivenza nell'Infarto-1 study. The GISSI Investigators. *Circulation*, 1998 Dec 15;98(24):2659–65.

[151] Baigent C, Collins R, Appleby P, Parish S, Sleight P, Peto R. ISIS-2: 10 year survival among patients with suspected acute myocardial infarction in randomised comparison of intravenous streptokinase, oral aspirin, both, or neither. The ISIS-2 (Second International Study of Infarct Survival) Collaborative Group. *BMJ*, 1998 May 2;316(7141):1337–43.

[152] Califf RM, White HD, Van de Werf F, Sadowski Z, Armstrong PW, Vahanian A, et al. One-year results from the Global Utilization of Streptokinase and TPA for Occluded Coronary Arteries (GUSTO-I) trial. GUSTO-I Investigators. *Circulation*, 1996 Sep 15;94(6):1233–8.

[153] Smalling RW, Bode C, Kalbfleisch J, Sen S, Limbourg P, Forycki F, et al. More rapid, complete, and stable coronary thrombolysis with bolus administration of reteplase compared with alteplase infusion in acute myocardial infarction. RAPID Investigators. *Circulation*, 1995 Jun 1;91(11):2725–32.

[154] Bode C, Smalling RW, Berg G, Burnett C, Lorch G, Kalbfleisch JM, et al. Randomized comparison of coronary thrombolysis achieved with double-bolus reteplase (recombinant plasminogen activator) and front-

loaded, accelerated alteplase (recombinant tissue plasminogen activator) in patients with acute myocardial infarction. The RA. *Circulation,* 1996 Sep 1;94(5):891–8.

[155] A comparison of reteplase with alteplase for acute myocardial infarction. The Global Use of Strategies to Open Occluded Coronary Arteries (GUSTO III) Investigators. *N. Engl. J. Med.,* 1997 Oct 16;337(16): 1118–23.

[156] Topol EJ, Ohman EM, Armstrong PW, Wilcox R, Skene AM, Aylward P, et al. Survival outcomes 1 year after reperfusion therapy with either alteplase or reteplase for acute myocardial infarction: results from the Global Utilization of Streptokinase and t-PA for Occluded Coronary Arteries (GUSTO) III Trial. *Circulation,* 2000 Oct 10;102(15):1761–5.

[157] Randomised, double-blind comparison of reteplase double-bolus administration with streptokinase in acute myocardial infarction (INJECT): trial to investigate equivalence. International Joint Efficacy Comparison of Thrombolytics. *Lancet,* 1995 Aug 5;346(8971):329–36.

[158] Keyt BA, Paoni NF, Refino CJ, Berleau L, Nguyen H, Chow A, et al. A faster-acting and more potent form of tissue plasminogen activator. *Proc. Natl. Acad. Sci. USA,* 1994 Apr 26;91(9):3670–4.

[159] Cannon CP, McCabe CH, Gibson CM, Ghali M, Sequeira RF, McKendall GR, et al. TNK-tissue plasminogen activator in acute myocardial infarction. Results of the Thrombolysis in Myocardial Infarction (TIMI) 10A dose-ranging trial. *Circulation,* 1997 Jan 21;95(2):351–6.

[160] Cannon CP, Gibson CM, McCabe CH, Adgey AA, Schweiger MJ, Sequeira RF, et al. TNK-tissue plasminogen activator compared with front-loaded alteplase in acute myocardial infarction: results of the TIMI 10B trial. Thrombolysis in Myocardial Infarction (TIMI) 10B Investigators. *Circulation,* 98(25):2805–14.

[161] Van de Werf F, Cannon CP, Luyten A, Houbracken K, McCabe CH, Berioli S, et al. Safety assessment of single-bolus administration of TNK tissue-plasminogen activator in acute myocardial infarction: the ASSENT-1 trial. The ASSENT-1 Investigators. *Am. Heart J.,* 1999 May;137(5):786–91.

[162] Van de Werf F, Adgey J, Ardissino D, Armstrong PW, Aylward P, Barbash G, et al. Single-bolus tenecteplase compared with front-loaded alteplase in acute myocardial infarction: the ASSENT-2 double-blind randomised trial. *Lancet,* 1999 Aug 28;354(9180):716–22.

[163] den Heijer P, Vermeer F, Ambrosioni E, Sadowski Z, López-Sendón JL, von Essen R, et al. Evaluation of a weight-adjusted single-bolus plasminogen activator in patients with myocardial infarction: a double-blind, randomized angiographic trial of lanoteplase versus alteplase. *Circulation,* 1998 Nov 17;98(20):2117–25.

[164] Intravenous NPA for the treatment of infarcting myocardium early; InTIME-II, a double-blind comparison of single-bolus lanoteplase vs accelerated alteplase for the treatment of patients with acute myocardial infarction. *Eur. Heart J.,* 2000 Dec;21(24):2005–13.

[165] Topol EJ. Reperfusion therapy for acute myocardial infarction with fibrinolytic therapy or combination reduced fibrinolytic therapy and platelet glycoprotein IIb/IIIa inhibition: the GUSTO V randomised trial. *Lancet,* 2001 Jun 16;357(9272):1905–14.

[166] Savonitto S, Armstrong PW, Lincoff AM, Jia G, Sila CA, Booth J, et al. Risk of intracranial haemorrhage with combined fibrinolytic and glycoprotein IIb/IIIa inhibitor therapy in acute myocardial infarction. Dichotomous response as a function of age in the GUSTO V trial. *Eur. Heart J.,* 2003 Oct;24(20):1807–14.

[167] Efficacy and safety of tenecteplase in combination with enoxaparin, abciximab, or unfractionated heparin: the ASSENT-3 randomised trial in acute myocardial infarction. *Lancet,* 2001 Aug 25;358(9282):605–13.

[168] Lincoff AM, Califf RM, Van de Werf F, Willerson JT, White HD, Armstrong PW, et al. Mortality at 1 year with combination platelet glycoprotein IIb/IIIa inhibition and reduced-dose fibrinolytic therapy vs conventional fibrinolytic therapy for acute myocardial infarction: GUSTO V randomized trial. *JAMA,* 2002 Nov 6;288(17):2130–5.

[169] Gurm HS, Lincoff AM, Lee D, Tang WHW, Jia G, Booth JE, et al. Outcome of acute ST-segment elevation myocardial infarction in diabetics treated with fibrinolytic or combination reduced fibrinolytic therapy and platelet glycoprotein IIb/IIIa inhibition: lessons from the GUSTO V trial. *J. Am. Coll. Cardiol.,* 2004 Feb 18;43(4):542–8.

[170] Sinnaeve PR, Alexander JH, Bogaerts K, Belmans A, Wallentin L, Armstrong P, et al. Efficacy of tenecteplase in combination with enoxaparin, abciximab, or unfractionated heparin: one-year follow-up results of the Assessment of the Safety of a New Thrombolytic-3 (ASSENT-3) randomized trial in acute myocardial infarction. *Am. Heart J.,* 2004 Jun;147(6):993–8.

[171] Keeley EC, Boura JA, Grines CL. Primary angioplasty versus intravenous thrombolytic therapy for acute myocardial infarction: a

quantitative review of 23 randomised trials. *Lancet,* 2003 Jan 4;361(9351):13–20.

[172] Ross AM, Coyne KS, Moreyra E, Reiner JS, Greenhouse SW, Walker PL, et al. Extended mortality benefit of early postinfarction reperfusion. GUSTO-I Angiographic Investigators. Global Utilization of Streptokinase and Tissue Plasminogen Activator for Occluded Coronary Arteries Trial. *Circulation,* 1998 Apr 28;97(16):1549–56.

[173] Fernández-Avilés F, Alonso JJ, Peña G, Blanco J, Alonso-Briales J, López-Mesa J, et al. Primary angioplasty vs. early routine post-fibrinolysis angioplasty for acute myocardial infarction with ST-segment elevation: the GRACIA-2 non-inferiority, randomized, controlled trial. *Eur. Heart J.,* 2007 Apr;28(8):949–60.

[174] Danchin N, Coste P, Ferrières J, Steg P-G, Cottin Y, Blanchard D, et al. Comparison of thrombolysis followed by broad use of percutaneous coronary intervention with primary percutaneous coronary intervention for ST-segment-elevation acute myocardial infarction: data from the french registry on acute ST-elevation myocardial inf. *Circulation,* 2008 Jul 15;118(3):268–76.

[175] Primary versus tenecteplase-facilitated percutaneous coronary intervention in patients with ST-segment elevation acute myocardial infarction (ASSENT-4 PCI): randomised trial. *Lancet,* 2006 Feb 18;367(9510):569–78.

[176] Alp NJ, Gershlick AH, Carver A, Stevens SE, Wilcox R. Rescue angioplasty for failed thrombolysis in older patients: insights from the REACT trial. *Int. J. Cardiol.,* 2008 Apr 10;125(2):254–7.

[177] Gershlick AH, Stephens-Lloyd A, Hughes S, Abrams KR, Stevens SE, Uren NG, et al. Rescue angioplasty after failed thrombolytic therapy for acute myocardial infarction. *N. Engl. J. Med.,* 2005 Dec 29;353(26): 2758–68.

[178] Collet J-P, Montalescot G, Le May M, Borentain M, Gershlick A. Percutaneous coronary intervention after fibrinolysis: a multiple meta-analyses approach according to the type of strategy. *J. Am. Coll. Cardiol., 2006* Oct 3;48(7):1326–35.

[179] Wijeysundera HC, Vijayaraghavan R, Nallamothu BK, Foody JM, Krumholz HM, Phillips CO, et al. Rescue angioplasty or repeat fibrinolysis after failed fibrinolytic therapy for ST-segment myocardial infarction: a meta-analysis of randomized trials. *J. Am. Coll. Cardiol.,* 2007 Jan 30;49(4):422–30.

[180] Di Mario C, Dudek D, Piscione F, Mielecki W, Savonitto S, Murena E, et al. Immediate angioplasty versus standard therapy with rescue angioplasty after thrombolysis in the Combined Abciximab REteplase Stent Study in Acute Myocardial Infarction (CARESS-in-AMI): an open, prospective, randomised, multicentre trial. *Lancet,* 2008 Feb 16;371(9612):559–68.

[181] Cantor WJ, Fitchett D, Borgundvaag B, Ducas J, Heffernan M, Cohen EA, et al. Routine early angioplasty after fibrinolysis for acute myocardial infarction. *N. Engl. J. Med.,* 2009 Jun 25;360(26):2705–18.

[182] Fernandez-Avilés F, Alonso JJ, Castro-Beiras A, Vázquez N, Blanco J, Alonso-Briales J, et al. Routine invasive strategy within 24 hours of thrombolysis versus ischaemia-guided conservative approach for acute myocardial infarction with ST-segment elevation (GRACIA-1): a randomised controlled trial. *Lancet,* 364(9439):1045–53.

[183] Bøhmer E, Hoffmann P, Abdelnoor M, Arnesen H, Halvorsen S. Efficacy and safety of immediate angioplasty versus ischemia-guided management after thrombolysis in acute myocardial infarction in areas with very long transfer distances results of the NORDISTEMI (NORwegian study on DIstrict treatment of ST-elevation my. *J. Am. Coll. Cardiol.,* 2010 Jan 12;55(2):102–10.

[184] Scheller B, Hennen B, Hammer B, Walle J, Hofer C, Hilpert V, et al. Beneficial effects of immediate stenting after thrombolysis in acute myocardial infarction. *J. Am. Coll. Cardiol.,* 2003 Aug 20;42(4):634–41.

[185] Greenbaum AB, Grines CL, Bittl JA, Becker RC, Kereiakes DJ, Gilchrist IC, et al. Initial experience with an intravenous P2Y12 platelet receptor antagonist in patients undergoing percutaneous coronary intervention: results from a 2-part, phase II, multicenter, randomized, placebo- and active-controlled trial. *Am. Heart J.,* 2006 Mar;151 (3):689.e1–689.e10.

[186] Harrington RA, Stone GW, McNulty S, White HD, Lincoff AM, Gibson CM, et al. Platelet inhibition with cangrelor in patients undergoing PCI. *N. Engl. J. Med.,* 2009 Dec 10;361(24):2318–29.

[187] Bhatt DL, Lincoff AM, Gibson CM, Stone GW, McNulty S, Montalescot G, et al. Intravenous platelet blockade with cangrelor during PCI. *N. Engl. J. Med.,* 2009 Dec 10;361(24):2330–41.

[188] Leonardi S, Mahaffey KW, White HD, Gibson CM, Stone GW, Steg GW, et al. Rationale and design of the Cangrelor versus standard therapy to acHieve optimal Management of Platelet InhibitiON PHOENIX trial. *Am. Heart J.,* 2012 May;163(5):768–776.e2.

[189] Angiolillo DJ, Schneider DJ, Bhatt DL, French WJ, Price MJ, Saucedo JF, et al. Pharmacodynamic effects of cangrelor and clopidogrel: the platelet function substudy from the cangrelor versus standard therapy to achieve optimal management of platelet inhibition (CHAMPION) trials. *J. Thromb. Thrombolysis*, 2012 Jul;34(1):44–55.

[190] Angiolillo DJ, Firstenberg MS, Price MJ, Tummala PE, Hutyra M, Welsby IJ, et al. Bridging antiplatelet therapy with cangrelor in patients undergoing cardiac surgery: a randomized controlled trial. *JAMA*, 2012 Jan 18;307(3):265–74.

[191] Lee S-W, Park S-W, Kim Y-H, Yun S-C, Park D-W, Lee CW, et al. Drug-eluting stenting followed by cilostazol treatment reduces late restenosis in patients with diabetes mellitus the DECLARE-DIABETES Trial (A Randomized Comparison of Triple Antiplatelet Therapy with Dual Antiplatelet Therapy After Drug-Eluting Stent Im. *J. Am. Coll. Cardiol.*, 2008 Mar 25;51(12):1181–7.

[192] Lee S-W, Park S-W, Kim Y-H, Yun S-C, Park D-W, Lee CW, et al. Comparison of triple versus dual antiplatelet therapy after drug-eluting stent implantation (from the DECLARE-Long trial). *Am. J. Cardiol.*, 2007 Oct 1;100(7):1103–8.

[193] Tamhane U, Meier P, Chetcuti S, Chen K-Y, Rha S-W, Grossman MP, et al. Efficacy of cilostazol in reducing restenosis in patients undergoing contemporary stent based PCI: a meta-analysis of randomised controlled trials. *EuroIntervention*, 2009 Aug;5(3):384–93.

[194] Douglas JS, Holmes DR, Kereiakes DJ, Grines CL, Block E, Ghazzal ZMB, et al. Coronary stent restenosis in patients treated with cilostazol. *Circulation*, 2005 Nov 1;112(18):2826–32.

[195] Suh J-W, Lee S-P, Park K-W, Lee H-Y, Kang H-J, Koo B-K, et al. Multicenter randomized trial evaluating the efficacy of cilostazol on ischemic vascular complications after drug-eluting stent implantation for coronary heart disease: results of the CILON-T (influence of CILostazol-based triple antiplatelet therapy ON is. *J. Am. Coll. Cardiol.*, 2011 Jan 18;57(3):280–9.

[196] Lee S-W, Park S-W, Kim Y-H, Yun S-C, Park D-W, Lee CW, et al. A randomized, double-blind, multicenter comparison study of triple antiplatelet therapy with dual antiplatelet therapy to reduce restenosis after drug-eluting stent implantation in long coronary lesions: results from the DECLARE-LONG II (Drug-Eluting Sten. *J. Am. Coll. Cardiol.*, 2011 Mar 15;57(11):1264–70.

[197] Tricoci P, Huang Z, Held C, Moliterno DJ, Armstrong PW, Van de Werf F, et al. Thrombin-receptor antagonist vorapaxar in acute coronary syndromes. *N. Engl. J. Med.,* 2012 Jan 5;366(1):20–33.

[198] Mega JL, Braunwald E, Wiviott SD, Bassand J-P, Bhatt DL, Bode C, et al. Rivaroxaban in patients with a recent acute coronary syndrome. *N. Engl. J. Med.,* 2012 Jan 5;366(1):9–19.

[199] Cardiovascular and Renal Drugs Advisory Committee - Briefing Information for the May 23, 2012 Meeting of the Cardiovascular and Renal Drugs Advisory Committee [Internet]. Center for Drug Evaluation and Research; [cited 2012 Sep 4]. Available from: http://www.fda.gov/AdvisoryCommittees/CommitteesMeetingMaterials/Drugs/CardiovascularandRenalDrugsAdvisoryCommittee/ucm304754.htm

[200] Alexander JH, Lopes RD, James S, Kilaru R, He Y, Mohan P, et al. Apixaban with antiplatelet therapy after acute coronary syndrome. *N. Engl. J. Med., 2011* Aug 25;365(8):699–708.

In: Percutaneous Coronary Intervention
Editors: Huili Gan and Yujie Zhou
ISBN: 978-1-62618-962-1
© 2013 Nova Science Publishers, Inc.

*Chapter VI*

# Off-Pump Coronary Artery Bypass Surgery Is a Safe Revascularization Procedure for Left Main Coronary Artery Lesion—Our Experience

*Hui-li Gan,*[1,*] *Jian-qun Zhang,*[1] *Fang-jong Huang,*[1] *Cheng-xiong Gu,*[1] *Qing-yu Kong,*[1] *Xiong-rong Cao,*[1] *Ping Bo,*[1] *Pi-shan Wang,*[1] *Tong Liu*[2] *and Chun-shang Lu*[2]

[1]Cardiac Surgery Department, Beijing Anzhen Hospital, and Capital Medical University (BAZH—CMU), Beijing Institute of Heart, Lung and Blood Vessel Disease, Beijing, China
[3]Cardiology Department, Beijing Anzhen Hospital, and Capital Medical University (BAZH—CMU), Beijing Institute of Heart, Lung and Blood Vessel Disease, Beijing, China

* Corresponding author: Dr. Hui-li Gan, Cardiac Surgery Department, Beijing Anzhen Hospital, and Capital Medical University (BAZH—CMU), Beijing Institute of Heart, Lung and Blood Vessel Disease, Beijing 100029, China. Fax: 86-10-62244207; E-mail: ganhuili@ 126.com.

# Abstract

Objective: Our aim was to assess if left main coronary artery coronary stenosis (LMCA) lesion pose additional risk of early or mid-term mortality and /or major adverse cardiac and Cerebrovascular event (MACCE) after off pump coronary artery bypass grafting (OPCABG), as compared with non-left main coronary artery stenosis (Non-mainstem disease). Methods: From January 1, 2009 to December 31, 2010, 4869 patients had primary isolated OPCABG procedure at Beijing Anzhen Hospital. According to the pathology of left main coronary artery lesions, they were retrospectively classified as Non-mainstem disease group (n=3933), LMCA group (n=936). Propensity score were used to match the two groups, patients from Non-mainstem disease group (n=831) were randomly selected to match patients from LMCA group (n=831). Freedoms from MACCE of the two groups were calculated through Kaplan-Meier method. Results: the difference of the mortality, rates of MACCEs during the first 30 days between Non-mainstem disease group and LCAM group didn't reach any statistical significance (P=0.429, 0.127 respectively). With a mean follow-up of (12.8±7.5) months and a cumulative follow-up of 1769.6 patient–years, the difference of the freedom from MACCEs between two groups, calculated through Kaplan-Meier method, did not reach statistically significance also (P=0.831). Conclusion: the high volume OPCABG procedure in our single center proved that LMCA lesion does not pose additional early and mid-term risk to OPCABG. Therefore, so off-pump coronary artery bypass surgery is a safe revascularization procedure for left main coronary artery lesion.

Keywords: Coronary artery bypass grafting (CABG), left main coronary artery (LMCA)

# Introduction

Traditionally, left main coronary artery (LMCA) stenosis had been recognized as a risk factor for early death among patients undergoing coronary artery bypass grafting (CABG). [1-3] However, due to the improvement of the peri- and postoperative management of patients undergoing CABG, LMCA lesion no longer was a risk factor for early and late death after CABG. [4] According to current guidelines, CABG remains the treatment of choice for patients with severe coronary artery disease, including those with LMCA and those with three-vessel disease. [5, 6] In this era of drug-eluting stent (DES),

CABG remains the standard of care for patients with three-vessel or LMCA disease, since the use of CABG, as compared with PCI, resulted in lower rates of the combined end point of major adverse cardiac or Cerebrovascular events at 1 year. [7]

Off pump CABG (OPCABG) has now evolved as routine practice in some cardiac centers. However, the relative safety and efficacy of LMCA vs. non-left main coronary artery stenosis (Non-mainstem disease) lesions after OPCABG procedure need to been explored in large samples. Therefore, in this study, we evaluated the relative efficacy and safety of OPCABG between Non-mainstem disease and LMCA lesion. In order to correct the confounding factors and to decrease the selective bias, we used preoperative variables to match two groups and to allow for direct comparisons of outcomes during the first 30 days after the procedure and during the mid-term follow-up.

# Methods

## Study Design

From January 1, 2009 through December 31, 2010, 5323 patients had CABG procedure, of which 4869 (91.5 %) patients with previously untreated coronary artery disease had primary isolated OPCABG procedure, and 454 (8.5%) patients had on-pump CABG procedure, at the Beijing Anzhen Hospital. According to the pathology of LMCA, the 4869 OPCABG patients were retrospectively classified into Non-mainstem disease group (n=3933) or LMCA group (n=936). Non-mainstem disease group was defined as that the patients had coronary artery disease but without LMCA lesion. LMCA group was defined as that the patients had LMCA lesion with o/w other coronary artery lesion. Patients intended with primary on pump CABG (ONCABG) procedure, and concomitant valve or other cardiac surgery (e.g., mitral valve repair and ventricular aneurysm resection, et al.) (n=454 cases) were excluded from this study. The age ranged from 39 to 78 (mean 59.6±16.3) years old. The 454 patients with on-pump procedure, including primary on-pump CABG (ONCABG) procedure (n=65), concomitant valve replacement (n=231, of which, there were 83 aortic valve replacement, 113 mitral valve replacement, and 35 double valve replacement), left ventricular aneurysmectomy (n=51), mitral valve repair (n=74), tricuspid valve repair (n=17), aorta procedure (n=16, of which there were 6 Bentall procedure, 2 David procedure, and 8 ascending aorta replacement) were excluded from this study. Overall, 1253 patients (25.7%) had Canadian Cardiovascular Society (CCS) angina class IV symptoms. LMCA lesion was defined as at least 50% stenosis in LMCA. Table 1 presented the preoperative demographic characteristics and risk factors of the two groups.

We have calculated a propensity score for LMCA lesion to get match with similar clinical characteristics between the two groups. Logistic regression with backward selection was performed to calculate the propensity score. By matching propensity score, 831 patients from Non-mainstem disease group were randomly selected to match 831 patients from LMCA group. Preoperatively matched patients from Non-mainstem disease group served as a control group.

**Table 1. Preoperative Baseline Demographic Variables and Risk Factors in Non-mainstem disease Group and LMCA Group**

| Patient Demographics and Preoperative Risk Factors | Non-mainstem disease Group (n=3933) | LMCA Group (n=936) | $P$ (F or $\chi^2$) |
|---|---|---|---|
| Age, yrs | 63.8±12.5 | 60.4±10.6 | 0.000 (7.295) |
| Age older than 65, n (%) | 1717 (48.71) | 358 (43.5) | 0.001 (10.721) |
| SYNTAX scores | 25.1±15.2 | 28.±11.1 | 0.000 (5.576) |
| Female, n (%) | 1404 (35.8) | 356 (38.1) | 0.234 (1.419) |
| All type Diabetes mellitus, n (%) | 2187 (55.6) | 501 (53.6) | 0.286 (1.137) |
| Insulin-dependent DM, n (%) | 649 (16.4) | 145 (15.5) | 0.588 (0.293) |
| HSCRP (mg/L) | 4.9±1.9 | 4.8±1.7 | 0.162 (1.400) |
| Hyperlipidemia, n (%) | 3137 (79.8) | 728 (77.8) | 0.228 (1.455) |
| Current smoker, n (%) | 222 (56.5) | 501 (53.5) | 0.126 (2.342) |
| Renal insufficiency, n (%) | 311 (7.9) | 67 (7.2) | 0.575 (0.314) |
| Hypertension, n (%) | 2663 (67.7) | 638 (68.1) | 0.803 (0.062) |
| Family history of CAD, n (%) | 1349 (34.0) | 333 (35.6) | 0.416 (0.661) |
| Previous MI, n (%) | 1726 (43.9) | 424 (45.3) | 0.476 (0.509) |
| Peripheral vascular disease, n (%) | 326 (8.3) | 78 (8.3) | 0.953 (0.003) |
| LVEF<35 %, n (%) | 561 (14.3) | 127 (13.5) | 0.787 (0.48) |
| LVEF,% | 51.8±17.8 | 52.5±15.5 | 0.294 (1.051) |
| Congestive heart failure, n (%) | 585 (14.9) | 131 (14.0) | 0.861 (0.031) |

| Patient Demographics and Preoperative Risk Factors | Non-mainstem disease Group (n=3933) | LMCA Group (n=936) | P (F or χ2) |
|---|---|---|---|
| Transient ischemic attack, n (%) | 125 (3.2) | 29 (3.1) | 0.996 (0.000) |
| Stroke, n (%) | 188 (4.8) | 40 (4.3) | 0.569 (0.335) |
| Pulmonary disease, n (%) | 323 (8.2) | 70 (7.5) | 0.442 (0.592) |
| CCS angina class IV, n (%) | 897 (22.8) | 266 (28.5) | 0.001 (11.619) |
| Pre procedure IABP, n (%) | 48 (1.2) | 25 (2.7) | 0.005 (8.029) |
| Aspirin, n (%) | 3868 (98.3) | 929 (99.3) | 0.062 (3.492) |
| β-Blocker, n (%) | 3047 (77.5) | 735 (78.5) | 0.534 (387) |
| CCB, n (%) | 1728 (43.9) | 407 (43.5) | 0.862 (0.030) |
| Nitrates, n (%) | 3437 (87.4) | 819 (87.5) | 0.954 (0.003) |
| Statins, n (%) | 2589 (65.8) | 610 (65.2) | 0.780 (0.078) |
| EKG Diagnosis, n (%) | | | |
| Sinus rhythm, n (%) | 3682 (93.6) | 875 (93.5) | |
| Atrial fibrillation, n (%) | 216 (5.5) | 49 (5.2) | 0.701 (0.71) |
| Other rhythm, n (%) | 35 (0.9) | 12 (1.3) | |
| Enrollment diagnosis | | | |
| Silent ischemia, n (%) | 215 (5.5) | 46 (4.9) | |
| Stable angina, n (%) | 1462 (37.2) | 192 (20.5) | |
| Unstable angina, n (%) | 1962 (49.9) | 626 (66.9) | 0.000 (93.07) |
| Acute Myocardium infarction, n (%) | 294 (7.5) | 72 (7.7) | |
| Vessel territory with stenosis | | | |
| RCA, n (%) | 3693 (93.9) | 841 (89.9) | 0.000 (17.841) |
| LAD, n (%) | 3767 (95.8) | 936 (100) | 0.000 (35.129) |
| LCX, n (%) | 3639 (92.5) | 936 (100) | 0.000 (66.466) |
| Small LV aneurysm, n (%) | 457 (11.6) | 111 (11.9) | 0.902 (0.015) |

Non-mainstem disease Group: non-left main coronary artery stenosis group; LMCA Group: general left main coronary artery stenosis group; HSCRP: High-sensitive C-reactive protein; LMCA: left main coronary artery; LAD: left anterior descending artery; LCX: left circumflex artery; RCA: right coronary artery; CAD: coronary artery disease; CCS: Canadian Cardiovascular Society; stable angina was defined according to CCS system; unstable angina was classified according to the Braunwald classification. CCB: calcium channel blocker; LVEF: left ventricular ejection fraction; IABP: intra-aortic balloon pump; Value are means ± SD when appropriate. Small LV aneurysm was defined as LV aneurysm with a volume less than 20% of the left ventricle.

Angiographies were assessed for pathology of LMCA stenosis before the operation.

Table 2 presented the preoperative demographic characteristics and risk factors of the two groups after matching. After matching, patients in the two groups were well balanced with regard to most of the baseline demographic and clinical characteristics.

Also after the matching, the preprocedural rates of stroke, myocardial infarction, and IABP adoption were similar in the two groups.

The local ethics committee at Anzhen Hospital and Beijing Institute of Heart, Lung and Blood Vessel Diseases approved the use of clinical data for this study. Written informed consent was obtained from each patient for the surgical or interventional procedure.


## Procedure Techniques

Eight surgical teams affiliated to Anzhen Hospital performed all of the CABG procedures.

Since 2001, The strategy for all of the isolated CABG procedure in Anzhen Hospital were planed firstly to proceed as OPCABG procedure, only when the hemodynamic situation were unstable or could not sustain the off pump manipulation, the procedure would be switched into beating ONCABG procedure without clamping the aorta and hypothermia. All of the procedures were performed via a median sternotomy approach under general anesthesia, in which an Octopus stabilizer (Medtronics, US) was used for the distal anastamosis, and a Novare Enclose II manual proximal anastomotic device (Novare, US) was used for the proximal anamostasis.

If the planed OPCABG procedures were switched into beating ONCABG, in which a cardiopulmonary bypass (CPB) were installed, the distal and proximal anastamosis were also completed with the aid of Octopus stabilizer and Novare Enclose II manual proximal anastomotic device.

The distal anastamosis were constructed with a continuous running 7-0 or 8-0 polypropylene suture and the proximal vein anastamosis to the aorta sutured over a partially secluded area in aorta by Novare Enclose II manual proximal anastomotic device with a continuous running 6-0 polypropylene suture.

All patients in the two groups were advised to continue lifelong aspirin therapy (100 mg daily).

**Table 2. Preoperative Baseline Demographic Variables and Risk Factors in the Non-mainstem disease, LMCA Group after Matching**

| Patient Demographics and Preoperative Risk Factors | Non-mainstem disease Group (n=831) | LMCA Group (n=831) | $P$ (F or $\chi^2$) |
|---|---|---|---|
| Age, yrs | 59.5±11.4 | 58.6±10.3 | 0.092 (0.533) |
| Age older than 65, n | 345 | 357 | 0.586 (0.298) |
| SYNTAX scores | 28.6±9.4 | 28.9±9.5 | 0.518 (0.647) |
| Female, n | 357 | 342 | 0.487 (0.484) |
| All type Diabetes mellitus, n | 421 | 400 | 0.367 (0.963) |
| Insulin-dependent DM, n | 141 | 133 | 0.644 (0.213) |
| HSCRP (mg/L) | 4.5±2.1 | 4.4±2.2 | 0.343 (0.948) |
| Hyperlipidemia, n | 637 | 627 | 0.605 (0.208) |
| Current smoker, n | 432 | 436 | 0.883 (0.022) |
| Renal insufficiency, n | 76 | 71 | 0.730 (0.119) |
| Hypertension, n | 584 | 581 | 0.915 (0.011) |
| Family history of CAD, n | 324 | 327 | 0.920 (0.010) |
| Previous MI, n | 410 | 418 | 0.731 (0.118) |
| Peripheral vascular disease, n | 65 | 68 | 0.857 (0.033) |
| LVEF < 35 %, n | 108 | 101 | 0.684 (0.166) |
| LVEF, % | 53.5±16.4 | 53.2±17.4 | 0.718 (0.362) |
| Congestive heart failure, n | 130 | 121 | 0.587 (0.295) |
| Transient ischemic attack, n | 43 | 43 | 1 (0) |
| Stroke, n | 33 | 32 | 0.899 (0.016) |
| Pulmonary disease, n | 87 | 79 | 0.567 (0.328) |
| CCS angina class IV | 328 | 336 | 0.726 (0.123) |
| Pre procedure IABP | 19 | 24 | 0.537 (0.382) |
| Aspirin, n | 831 | 829 | 0.479 (0.501) |
| β-Blocker, n | 724 | 715 | 0.093 (2.827) |
| CCB, n | 389 | 379 | 0.658 (0.196) |
| Nitrates, n | 756 | 763 | 0.600 (0.275) |
| Statins, n | 519 | 548 | 0.152 (2.052) |
| EKG Diagnosis | | | |
| Sinus rhythm, n | 766 | 769 | |
| Atrial fibrillation, n | 54 | 53 | 0.896 (0.22) |
| Other rhythm, n | 11 | 9 | |

**Table 2. (Continued)**

| Patient Demographics and Preoperative Risk Factors | Non-mainstem disease Group (n=831) | LMCA Group (n=831) | $P$ (F or $\chi^2$) |
|---|---|---|---|
| Enrollment diagnosis, | | | |
| Silent ischemia, n | 42 | 38 | |
| Stable angina, n | 176 | 171 | |
| Unstable angina, n | 548 | 559 | 0.920 (0.01) |
| Acute myocardium infarction, n | 65 | 63 | |
| Vessel territory with stenosis | | | |
| RCA, n | 748 | 747 | 0.901 (0.016) |
| LAD | 831 | 831 | 1 (0) |
| LCX | 831 | 831 | 1 (0) |
| Small LV aneurysm | 98 | 93 | 0.758 (0.095) |

Non-mainstem disease Group: non-left main coronary artery stenosis group; LMCA Group: general left main coronary artery stenosis group; HSCRP: High-sensitive C-reactive protein; LMCA: left main coronary artery; LAD: left anterior descending artery; LCX: left circumflex artery; RCA: right coronary artery; CAD: coronary artery disease; CCS: Canadian Cardiovascular Society; stable angina was defined according to CCS system; unstable angina was classified according to the Braunwald classification. CCB: calcium channel blocker; LVEF: left ventricular ejection fraction; IABP: intra-aortic balloon pump; Value are means ± SD when appropriate. Small LV aneurysm was defined as LV aneurysm with a volume less than 20% of the left ventricle.

## Study Endpoints

The primary endpoint was all cause mortality within 30 days after the revascularization procedure and during the follow-up. The secondary endpoint was the incidence of major adverse cardiac and cerebrovascular events (MACCEs) within 30 days after the revascularization procedure and during the follow-up. MACCEs were defined as all-cause death, nonfatal myocardial infarction, stroke and repeated revascularization. Repeated revascularization was defined as any percutaneous coronary intervention (PCI) or bypass surgery after the first revascularization procedure. Non-Q-wave myocardial infarction was diagnosed according to World Health Organization criteria, including an increase in total creatine kinase (CK) level to ≥2× the upper limit of the normal range and an elevated MB isoform level without development of new pathological Q waves. A Q-wave myocardial infarction was present when, in addition to CK elevation, a new pathological Q wave was noted in at least two leads.

## Data Collection

One month after discharge, all surviving patients from two groups were assessed at an outpatient clinic for full review by the cardiac surgeon or cardiologist. CCS angina class, troponin (Tn)-I and cardiac enzymes, transthoracic echocardiography (TTE) and ECG data were recorded. These variables were evaluated at 3-month intervals. Long-term clinical outcomes were assessed up to July 2011 by reviewing the medical files of their cardiologists or general practitioners, or both, when appropriate. Baseline demographics, procedural data and perioperative outcomes were recorded. For deaths after the first 30 days post the CABG procedure, the medical files were reviewed by one of the primary investigators of this study. The status of the patients was determined by review of hospital records, follow-up questionnaires, or contact with local physicians at an interval of 3 months after the first outpatient visit. Detailed information, including CCS angina class status, cardiac rhythm, complications and present medications were recorded. At the follow-up, TTE and ECG were assessed in 1612 (98.5%) of the 1636 patients surviving hospitalization and the main parameters were collected. Twenty-three of our patients were lost to follow-up. Patient demographics, preoperative risk factors and the incidence of adverse postoperative outcomes were retrieved from the Digitalcare database at Anzhen Hospital. Diagnostic angiograms were scored, according to the SYNTAX score algorithm [8] by one investigator of this study.

## Statistical Analysis

All statistical analyses were performed with the statistical software package SPSS 17.0 (SPSS Inc., an IBM Company, Chicago, Ill). Most continuous variables were presented as mean ± standard deviation (mean ± SD). Categorical data were summarized as frequencies and percentages. Cumulative event rates such as freedom from MACCEs of the two groups were estimated by means of the Kaplan–Meier method.

Differences among patients of two groups were analyzed with one-way ANOVA, interactive Chi-square tests [9], Fisher's exact test, or Wilcoxon rank sum tests, or Log rank test as appropriate.

# Results

## Revascularization Data

The results were focused on the two matched groups. The average interval between the diagnostic angiogram and the CABG procedure was 11.3 ± 4.9 days. Because of the unstable hemodynamic situation during the intended off pump manipulation, there were 19 (2.25%), 22 (2.61%) conversion to ONCABG from OPCABG in Non-mainstem disease, LMCA group respectively, so the difference of the rate of conversion to cardiopulmonary bypass between two groups did not reached statistically significance ($\chi^2$=0.225, P=0.635). The mean distal anastamosis in LMCA group (3.46 ± 0.93) was similar to that in Non-mainstem disease group (3.54 ±0.89), (t=1.568, P=0.117). In all of the patients in Non-mainstem disease group, at least one arterial conduit was used, including the left internal mammary artery (LIMA) in 820 (98.6%) of the patients, bilateral internal mammary artery in 39 (4.63%) of patients, and radial artery grafts in 48 (5.69%) patients. In all of the patients in LMCA group, at least one arterial conduit was used, including the left internal mammary artery (LIMA) in 818(98.4%) of the patients, bilateral internal mammary artery in 21(2.49%) of patients, and radial artery grafts in 29 (3.44%) patients. So the difference of the rate of arterial conduit usage between two groups did not reached statistically significance ($\chi^2$= 1.231, P=0.367). There were 18 (2.14%), 22 (2.61%) patients in Non-mainstem disease, LMCA group respectively who adopted intra-aortic balloon pump (IABP) during perioperative period, and the difference of the rate of IABP use among two groups did not reach statistically significance ($\chi^2$= 0.410, P=0.522).

## Outcomes during the First 30 Days

The results were focused on the two matched groups. As presented in table 3, the difference of the mortality during the first 30 days between Non-mainstem disease group (1.32 %) and LCAM group (1.81%) did not reached statistically significance. ($\chi^2$=0.625, P=0.429). The OR (95% CI) of LCAM vs. Non-mainstem disease is 1.37 (0.63–3.00).

**Table 3. Clinical End Points Within First 30 Days after the
Revascularization and During Follow-up**

| MACCE (%) | Non-mainstem disease Group | LMCA Group | OR (95% CI) | $P$ ($\chi^2$) |
|---|---|---|---|---|
| First 30 days | | | | |
| No. of patients | (n=831) | (n=831) | | |
| Death | 11 (1.32%) | 15 (1.81%) | 1.37 (0.63–3.00) | 0.429 (0.625) |
| Myocardium infarction | 26 (3.12 %) | 32 (3.85%) | 1.24 (0.73–2.10) | 0.423 (0.643) |
| Stroke | 15 (1.81%)· | 16 (1.93%) | 1.07 (0.53–2.18) | 0.856 (0.033) |
| Death/myocardium infarction/stroke | 52 (6.26%) | 63 (7.58%) | 1.23 (0.84–1.80) | 0.288 (1.130) |
| Redo-CABG | 3 (0.36%) | 4 (0.48%) | 1.35 (0.30–5.98) | 0.705 (0.143) |
| Redo-PCI | 4 (0.48%) | 9 (1.08%) | 2.26 (0.69–7.38) | 0.164 (1.938) |
| Repeat revascularization | 7 (0.84 %) | 13 (1.54%) | 1.87 (0.74–4.71) | 0.177 (1.822) |
| Any MACCE | 59 (7.09%) | 76 (9.15%) | 1.32 (0.92–1.88) | 0.127 (2.330) |
| Mid-term follow-up | | | | |
| No. of patients | 820 | 816 | | |
| Death | 8 (0.86%) | 10 (1.30%) | 1.25 (0.49–3.19) | 0.682 (0.235) |
| Myocardium infarction | 22 (2.68%) | 25 (3.63%) | 1.14 (0.64–2.04) | 0.645 (0.213) |
| Stroke | 29 (3.54%) | 28 (3.43%) | 0.96 (0.57–1.64) | 0.575 (0.314) |
| Death/myocardium infarction/stroke | 59 (7.20%) | 63 (7.72%) | 1.07 (0.74–1.55) | 0.686 (0.164) |
| Redo-CABG | 0 (0%) | 0 (0%) | Na | 1 |
| Redo-PCI | 8 (0.98%) | 11 (1.35%) | 1.38 (0.55–3.45) | 0.482 (0.494) |
| Repeat revascularization | 8 (0.98%) | 11 (1.35%) | 1.38 (0.55–3.45) | 0.678 (0.172) |
| Any MACCE | 67 (8.17%) | 74 (9.07%) | 1.12 (0.79–1.57) | 0.518 (0.419) |

The difference of the rate of MACCE during the first 30 days between Non-mainstem disease group (7.09%) and LCAM group (9.15%) did not reached statistically significance. ($\chi^2$= 2.330, $P$=0.127). The OR (95% CI) of Non-mainstem disease vs. LMCA is 1.32 (0.92–1.88).

## Clinical Follow-Up

Of the 1636 survivors from the two groups, twenty-three of our patients were lost to follow up, so Follow-up was completed in 98.6%.

The mean follow-up was (12.8±7.5) Months, with a range of 1 to 26 months and the cumulated follow-up were 1769.6 patient–years. As presented in Table 3, the difference of the incidence of MACCE during follow-up between Non-mainstem disease group (8.17 %) and LMCA group (9.07%) did not reached statistically significance ($\chi^2$= 0.419, P=0.518). The difference of the freedom from MACCE between two groups, calculated through Kaplan-Meier method, did not reached statistically significance also ($\chi^2$=0.460, P=0.831) (Figure 1 and Table 4).

# Discussion

Coronary artery bypass grafting was first performed without the use of cardiopulmonary bypass (CPB) in the late 1960s, [10] but this technique was largely abandoned after the use of CPB and cardioplegic arrest became routine. [11]

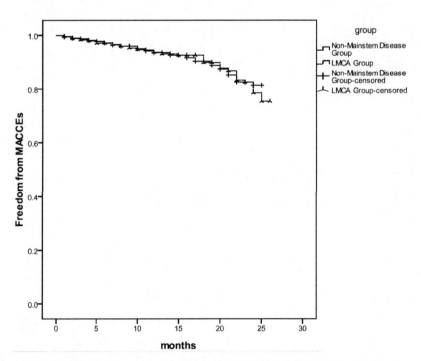

Figure 1. The Kaplan-Meier curves of freedom from MACCEs for Non-mainstem Disease Group, LMCA Group.

**Table 4. Freedom from MACCEs for Non-mainstem disease, LMCA
Group after Correction (%)**

|  | Non-mainstem disease Group | LMCA Group | P* value ($\chi^2$) |
|---|---|---|---|
| 12 months | 93.6±1.0 | 93.7±1.0 | |
| 18 months | 88.8±1.6 | 89.9±1.4 | 0.831 (0.46) |
| 24 months | 81.3±2.6 | 75.4±3.6 | |

*Log-rank test for Kaplan-Meier MACCE-free curve between Non-mainstem disease
and LMCA group.

However, as coronary revascularization methods continue to be refined, and OPCABG technique was one of major progresses in this field, it has evolved as a routine practice in some cardiac centers such as ours.

OPCABG can achieve with a low mortality and good medium to long-term survival. OPCABG is associated with fewer post-op complications and comparable late coronary interventions. [12] A modern OPCABG approach offers low mortality, excellent clinical outcomes, and does not come at the price of less complete revascularization in the high-risk patient. [13] OPCABG appears to reduce length of hospital stay, operative morbidity, and operative mortality relative to ONCABG. Although more studies are required before firm conclusions can be drawn concerning the effect of OPCABG on mid-term or long-term mortality, angina recurrence, and repeat intervention [14], OPCABG results in better preservation of left ventricular function in the perioperative period than conventional ONCABG. [15]

Risk factors associated with increased operative mortality post-CABG for severe LMCA disease are slightly different from those identified for CABG for all atherosclerotic disease. In addition to female sex, older age and left ventricular impairment, studies have identified additional specific risk factors for operative mortality in CABG for LMCA disease, including Canadian Cardiovascular Society anginal scores III—IV, duration of anginal symptoms, left dominant coronary artery anatomy, increased duration of cardiopulmonary bypass time, fewer grafts, [16] significant right coronary artery stenosis and absence of collaterals. [17]

Therefore, significant LMCA stenosis is a consistent predictor of morbidity and mortality after CABG. Low cardiac output states are significantly more common post-CABG in patients with significant LMCA disease. [18] The Society of Thoracic Surgeons database shows a relative risk of perioperative mortality of 1.3 for patients with significant LMCA stenosis, compared with patients without LMCA disease.

At 5 years post-CABG, the mortality in patients with three-vessel disease is 10.7%, compared with 15.8% in patients with LMCA disease. [19] Therefore, LMCA disease is an important independent risk factor for increased mortality and morbidity at all stages of diagnosis and treatment of coronary artery disease. Although there have been advances in the percutaneous treatment of LMCA stenosis resulting in indications for PCI in clearly defined patient groups with LMCA disease, CABG confers a significant event-free survival benefit over percutaneous and medical treatment in high- and low-risk patient subsets, that persists over 15 years postoperatively. Despite advances in the diagnosis and management of these patients, LMCA disease remains a poor prognostic factor. Therefore, the presence of critical left LMCA disease was, until recently, considered a relative contraindication to the use of off-pump techniques.

However, haemodynamic disturbances during displacement of the heart have been minimised, thanks to improvements in stabiliser technology, use of intra-coronary shunts and greater surgical and, perhaps most importantly, anaesthetic experience. A meta-analysis of nine studies comparing outcomes of on- and off-pump surgery in patients with severe LMCA disease in 4411 patients showed a statistically significant reduction in the rates of post-operative stroke in the off-pump groups than in on-pump groups. [20] Despite greater preoperative co-morbidity, including a higher incidence of poor left ventricular function in the off-pump groups than in the on-pump groups, these studies consistently showed equivalent or improved out-comes in patients treated with off-pump surgery. Perioperative mortality ranged from 0.0% to 1.9% in the off-pump group compared with 2.2% to 6% with conventional CABG. Although in three of these studies off-pump patients received significantly fewer grafts, it is difficult to assess whether this was due to clinical or technical reasons as none of the studies was randomized.

There was a pronounced decrease of the risk of both early and late death during the last decade in patients with LMCA disease undergoing CABG. During this long period, there were major improvements within almost all fields regarding perioperative management of patients undergoing open-heart surgery. These cumulative beneficial effects of continuous advancement in operative, anesthetic and medical management all contributed to the improved survival. [21, 22] Møller CH [23] reported that both off- and on-pump coronary artery bypass grafting could be performed in high-risk patients with low short-term complications.

In the era of DES, CABG remains the method of choice for patients with LMCA disease. [5, 6, 7]

According to experience from the Cleveland Clinic Foundation, left main disease was completely neutralized as a risk factor for operative mortality.[24] Once a time, significant LMCA stenosis (> or =50%) has been considered a relative contraindication to OPCABG, stemming from well-documented hemodynamic perturbations during the displacement of the heart. However, Beauford and his collegues proved that multi-vessel off-pump revascularization in patients with severe LMCA disease is a safe and effective alternative to conventional bypass grafting and conveys a survival benefit. [25] Yeatman also demonstrated that OPCAB is safe and effective in patients with critical LMCA disease in terms of early and late mortality and MACCE events. [26] Suzuki and his colleagues have also demonstrated the safety of performing OPCABG surgery in all patients, without the use of exclusion criteria. Early and mid-term outcomes were acceptable and encouraged continued use of the OPCABG approach in all CABG patients. [27] Karic and his colleagues revealed that OPCAB is effective and safe method for treatment of LMCA lesion, and there are certain advantages in comparison to classical method in short-term follow-up, with no difference in long-term results. [28] Panesar and his colleagues demonstrated that OPCABG might offer a neurological benefit in patients with significant LMCA disease undergoing CABG. [29]

However, all of the above literatures were small series report, and none of them explored the early and medium to long-term outcomes after OPCABG procedure to LMCA leasions in a large volume of subjects, thus leave much room of uncertainty for their conclusion. High volume experience in OPCABG treating LMCA lesion are needed to provide further and more convincible evidence. Through the last 10 years off-pump coronary artery bypass (OPCAB) surgery has constantly gained popularity in the cardiovascular community. Now accounting for 20% of the coronary artery bypass grafting (CABG) practice in the US and probably up to 15% in Canada, its use is expected to grow. In our hospital, Beijing Anzhen Hospital, the OPCAB accounted about 85% of the CABG procedure. Our cardiac center performed a high volume of CABG procedures each year, which reached 2900 cases in 2011. In our center, off-pump CABG had been performed regularly for more than 10 years before the launch of the trial and each of our surgical teams have performed at least 85% of their isolated CABG as off-pump procedures since 2005. In our series of single center, LMCA account about 18% of the CABG population. Therefore, our high volume clinical practice in revascularization procedure provided a more convincible basis to analyze the early and mid to long-term effect of OPCAB procedure to LMCA lesions.

Our study proved that Off-pump surgery offers equivalent outcomes to for LMCA disease as compared with Non-mainstem disease.

## Study Limitations

This study is a retrospective analysis and some confounding factors may hide any clear association between the early and late prognoses of OPCABG and the pathology of LMCA lesion. Although we used matching to balance the two non-equivalent groups and reduce any bias for a specific revascularization procedure, prospective randomized comparative trials are needed to confirm the findings of this study. However, the large volume of our research subjects in single center still could provide a basis for our conclusion.

## Conclusion

Our single center experiences proves that high volume OPCABG procedure in our single center proved that LMCA lesion does not pose additional early and mid-term risk to OPCABG. Therefore, Therefore, so off-pump coronary artery bypass surgery is a safe revascularization procedure for theleft main coronary artery lesion.

## References

[1]    Hannan, E. L., Kilburn, Jr. H., O'Donnell, J. F., Lukacik, G., Shields, E. P. Adult open heart surgery in New York State. An analysis of risk factors and hospital mortality rates. *J. Am. Med. Assoc.* 1990;264:2768-74.

[2]    Davierwala, P. M., Maganti, M., Yau, T. M. Decreasing significance of left ventricular dysfunction and reoperative surgery in predicting coronary artery bypass grafting-associated mortality: a twelve-year study. *J. Thorac. Cardiovasc. Surg.* 2003; 126:1335-44.

[3]    Jones, R. H., Hannan, E. L., Hammermeister, K. E., Delong, E. R., O'Connor, G. T., Luepker, R. V., Parsonnet, V., Pryor, D. B, The Working Group Panel on the Cooperative CABG Database Project Identification of preoperative variables needed for risk adjustment of

short-term mortality after coronary artery bypass graft surgery. *J. Am. Coll. Cardiol.* 1996;28:1478-87.

[4]     Jönsson, A., Hammar, N., Nordquist, T., Ivert, T. Left main coronary artery stenosis no longer a risk factor for early and late death after coronary artery bypass surgery--an experience covering three decades. *Eur. J. Cardiothorac. Surg.* 2006; 30:311-7.

[5]     Smith, S. C. Jr, Feldman, T. E., Hirshfeld, J. W. Jr, et al. ACC/AHA/SCAI 2005 guideline update for percutaneous coronary intervention: a report of the American College of Cardiology/American Heart Association Task Force on Practice Guidelines (ACC/AHA/SCAI Writing Committee to Update the 2001 Guidelines for Percutaneous Corona r y Inter vent ion). *J. Am. Coll. Cardiol.* 2006; 47:e1-e121.

[6]     Anderson, J. L., Adams, C. D., Antman, E. M., Bridges, C. R., Califf, R. M., Casey, D. E. Jr, et al. ACC/AHA 2007 guidelines for the management of patients with unstable angina/non-ST-Elevation myocardial infarction: a report of the American College of Cardiology/ American Heart Association Task Force on Practice Guidelines (Writing Committee to Revise the 2002 Guidelines for the Management of Patients With Unstable Angina/Non-ST-Elevation Myocardial Infarction) developed in collaboration with the American College of Emergency Physicians, the Society for Cardiovascular Angiography and Interventions, and the Society of Thoracic Surgeons endorsed by the American Association of Cardiovascular and Pulmonary Rehabilitation and the Society for Academic Emergency Medicine. *J. Am. Coll. Cardiol.* 2007;50(7):e1-e157.

[7]     Serruys, P. W., Morice, M. C., Kappetein, A. P., Colombo, A., Holmes, D. R., Mack, M. J., et al. Percutaneous coronary intervention versus coronary-artery bypass grafting for severe coronary artery disease. *N Engl. J. Med.* 2009;360:961-72.

[8]     Sianos, G., Morel, M. A., Kappetein, A. P., et al. The SYNTAX score: an angiographic tool grading the complexity of coronary artery disease. *Euro. Intervention.* 2005; 1: 219-27.

[9]     Preacher, K. J. (2001, April). Calculation for the chi-square test: An interactive calculation tool for chi-square tests of goodness of fit and independence [Computer software]. Available from http://www. quantpsy.org.

[10]    Kirklin, J. K., Westaby, S., Blackstone, E. H., Kirklin, J. W., Chenoweth, D. E., Pacifico, A. D. Complement and the damaging

effects of cardiopulmonary bypass. *J. Thorac. Cardiovasc. Surg.* 1983; 86(6):845-57.

[11]   Buffolo, E., Andrade, C. S., Branco, J. N., Teles, C. A., Aguiar, L. F., Gomes, W. J. Coronary arteries bypass grafting without cardiopulmonary bypass. *Ann. Thorac. Surg.* 1996;61(1):63-6.

[12]   Nwaejike, N., Mansha, M., Bonde, P., Campalani, G. Myocardial revascularization by off pump coronary bypass surgery (OPCABG): a ten year review. *Ulster. Med. J.* 2008; 77:106-9.

[13]   Emmert, M. Y., Salzberg, S. P., Seifert, B., Schurr, U. P., Hoerstrup, S. P., Reuthebuch, O., et al. Routine off-pump coronary artery bypass grafting is safe and feasible in high-risk patients with left main disease. *Ann. Thorac. Surg.* 2010;89:1125-30.

[14]   Reston, J. T., Tregear, S. J., Turkelson, C. M. Meta-analysis of short-term and mid-term outcomes following off-pump coronary artery bypass grafting. *Ann. Thorac. Surg.* 2003; 76:1510-5.

[15]   Pegg, T. J., Selvanayagam, J. B., Karamitsos, T. D., Arnold, R. J., Francis, J. M., Neubauer, S., et al. Effects of off-pump versus on-pump coronary artery bypass grafting on early and late right ventricular function. *Circulation.* 2008; 117:2202-10.

[16]   Chaitman, B. R., Rogers, W. J., Davis, K., Tyras, D. H., Berger, R., Bourassa, M. G., Fisher, L., Stover Hertzberg, V., Judkins, M. P., Mock, M. B., Killip, T. Operative risk factors in patients with left main coronary-artery disease. *N Engl. J. Med.* 1980;303:953—7.

[17]   Shen, A. Y., Jandhyala, R., Ruel, C., Lundstrom, R. J., Jorgensen, M. B. Predictors of survival after coronary bypass grafting in patients with total occlusion of the left main coronary artery. *Am. J. Cardiol.* 1998;81: 343—6.

[18]   Rao, V., Ivanov, J., Weisel, R. D., Ikonomidis, J. S., Christakis, G. T., David, T. E. Predictors of low cardiac output syndrome after coronary artery bypass. *J. Thorac. Cardiovasc. Surg.* 1996;112:38—51.

[19]   Keogh, B. E., Kinsman, R. Fifth national adult cardiac surgical database report 2003. Improving outcomes for patients. The Society of Cardiothoracic Surgeons of Great Britain and Ireland. Oxfordshire UK: Dendrite Clinical Systems; 2003.

[20]   Panesar, S. S., Chikwe, J., Mirza, S. B., Rahman, M. S., Warren, O., Rao, C., Negus, J., Zacharakis, E., Darzi, A., Athanasiou, T. Off-pump coronary artery bypass surgery may reduce the incidence of stroke in patients with significant left main stem disease. *Thorac. Cardiovasc. Surg.* 2008;56:247—55.

[21] Abramov, D., Tamariz, M. G., Fremes, S. E., Guru, V., Borger, M. A., Christakis, G. T., Bhatnagar, G., Sever, J. Y., Goldman, B. S. Trends in coronary artery bypass surgery results: a recent, 9-year study. *Ann. Thorac. Surg.* 2000; 70:84-90.

[22] Pryor, D. B., Harrell, Jr. F. E., Rankin, J. S., Lee, K. L., Muhlbaier, L. H., Oldham, H. N., Hlatky, M. A., Mark, D. B., Reves, J. G., Califf, R. M. The changing survival benefits of coronary revascularization over time. *Circulation* 1987; 76:V13-V21.

[23] Møller, C. H., Perko, M. J., Lund, J. T., Andersen, L. W., Kelbaek, H., Madsen, J. K., Winkel, P., Gluud, C., Steinbrüchel, D. A. No major differences in 30-day outcomes in high-risk patients randomized to off-pump versus on-pump coronary bypass surgery: the best bypass surgery trial. *Circulation.* 2010;121(4):498-504.

[24] Cosgrove, D. M., Loop, F. D., Lytle, B. W., Baillot, R., Gill, C. C., Golding, L. A., et al. Primary myocardial revascularization. Trends in surgical mortality. *J. Thorac. Cardiovasc. Surg.* 1984;/88:/673-84.

[25] Beauford, R. B., Saunders, C. R., Lunceford, T. A., Niemeier, L. A., Shah, S., Karanam, R., et al. Multivessel off-pump revascularization in patients with significant left main coronary artery stenosis: early and midterm outcome analysis. *J. Card. Surg.* 2005; 20:112-8.

[26] Yeatman, M., Caputo, M., Ascione, R., Ciulli, F., Angelini, G. D. Off-pump coronary artery bypass surgery for critical left main stem disease: safety, efficacy and outcome. *Eur. J. Cardiothorac. Surg.* 2001;19:239-44.

[27] Suzuki, T., Asai, T. Early and midterm results of off-pump coronary artery bypass grafting without patient selection. *Heart Surg. Forum.* 2008;11:E213-7.

[28] Karic, A., Mujanovic, E., Karic, A., Jerkic, Z., Bergsland, J., Kabil, E. Results of coronary bypass grafting in treatment of left main stenosis. *Med. Arh.* 2009;63:328-31

[29] Panesar, S. S., Chikwe, J., Mirza, S. B., Rahman, M. S., Warren, O., Rao, C., et al. Off-pump coronary artery bypass surgery may reduce the incidence of stroke in patients with significant left main stem disease. *Thorac. Cardiovasc. Surg.* 2008; 56:247-55.

In: Percutaneous Coronary Intervention          ISBN: 978-1-62618-962-1
Editors: Huili Gan and Yujie Zhou     © 2013 Nova Science Publishers, Inc.

*Chapter VII*

# Ostial Right Coronary Lesions: A Comparison between Percutaneous Coronary Intervention and Coronary Artery Bypass Grafts Adjusted by Propensity Score

*Hui-li Gan*[\*,1] *, Tong Liu*[2]
*and Chun-shang Lu*[2]
[1]Cardiac Surgery Department,
[2]Cardiology Department,
Beijing Anzhen Hospital, Capital Medical University,
Beijing Institute of Heart,
Lung and Blood Vessel Disease, Beijing, China

[\*] Correspondence to: Dr. Hui-li Gan, Cardiac Surgery Department, Beijing Anzhen Hospital,
Capital Medical University (BAZH—CMU), Beijing Institute of Heart, Lung and Blood
Vessel Disease, Beijing 100029, China (Fax: 86-10-62244207, Email:
ganhuili@hotmail.com).

# Abstract

Objective: Our aim was to evaluate the relative safety and efficacy of percutaneous coronary intervention (PCI) with drug-eluting stents (DES) versus coronary artery bypass grafts (CABG) for the treatment of ostial right coronary stenosis (ORCS) lesions.

Methods: 359 cases of ORCS lesion were treated via CABG (n=232) or PCI (n=127) procedures. Propensity scores for undergoing the CABG procedure were estimated and used to match 105 pairs of patients between the two groups. Kaplan-Meier major adverse cardiac and cerebrovascular events (MACCE)-free curves were constructed to compare long-term MACCE-free survival between the two groups.

Results: For the 105 propensity-matched pairs, patients were more likely to undergo PCI than CABG during the first 30 days (odds ratio [OR]: 2.040; 95% confidence interval [CI]: 1.78–2.27, P=0.043, $\chi^2$=4.08) and the late follow-up period (OR: 2.06; 95% CI: 1.79–2.38, P=0.02, $\chi^2$=5.17). With a mean follow-up of 12.04±6.47 months and a total of 210.67 patient–years, the freedom from MACCE in the CABG group was significantly higher than that in the PCI group (Log rank test, $\chi^2$=4.48, P=0.03). There were no significant differences in the rates of death, myocardial infarction, nonfatal stroke, death/myocardium infarction/stroke, or repeated PCI between the two groups during the first 30 days and during the late follow-up.

Conclusion: For OCRS lesions, CABG provided greater protection than PCI procedure in terms of freedom from MACCE, mainly due to the reduced number of repeated revascularization procedures. CABG should be considered as first-choice revascularization strategy for ORCS lesion.

# Introduction

Coronary artery ostial stenosis is an unusual manifestation of symptomatic coronary artery disease, and represents a challenge for interventional cardiologists because ostial atherosclerotic lesions are distinct from other lesion sites in terms of outcomes after percutaneous coronary intervention (PCI) [1].

Revascularization procedures, including coronary artery bypass grafts (CABG) and PCI, are associated with relatively high in-hospital and long-term mortality rates for patients with significant ostial right coronary stenosis (ORCS) disease.

However, the optimal revascularization strategy using either PCI or CABG in patients with ORCS lesions remain unclear. The introduction of antiproliferative drug-eluting stents (DES) has dramatically reduced the rates of restenosis and target lesion revascularization after PCI. However, despite low rates of in-hospital complications and the utilization of DES in most patients, the rate of major adverse cardiac and cerebrovascular events (MACCE) at 1 year remains high when compared with non-ostial proximal lesions. This increased mid-term risk must be considered by the surgeon.

Similarly, the possibility of performing CABG in patients with ORCS should also be considered before proceeding with PCI. However, the relative safety and efficacy of CABG and PCI for the revascularization of patients with ORCS has not been fully reported.

Because OCRS lesions were typically excluded or minimally represented in the earlier multicenter randomized trials that tested the efficacy of DES, the benefits of PCI and CABG have not been adequately evaluated [2]. Thus, it is unclear whether PCI with DES should be the preferred strategy for ORCS patient because of insufficient clinical evidence [3]. Therefore, in this study, we evaluated the relative efficacy and safety of CABG and PCI for revascularization in patients with ORCS in cohort of patients with ORCS treated between January 1, 2006 and December 31, 2007, at Anzhen Hospital. We used propensity score analysis to match the two groups and to allow for direct comparisons of outcomes during the first 30 days after the procedure and during a late follow-up period.

# Methods

## Study Design

This was a retrospective cohort study of patients who underwent primary CABG surgery or PCI (n=359) for ORCS lesions between January 1, 2006 and December 31, 2007 at Anzhen Hospital. ORCS was defined as stenosis of the proximal right coronary artery (less than 3 mm to the ostium of right coronary artery) of at least 75%. The primary inclusion criterion was for patients with ORCS lesions (n=359) who underwent PCI (n=232) or CABG (n=127). Patients with ORCS lesions and concomitant valve or other cardiac surgery (e.g., atrial septal defect repair and ventricular aneurysm resection) (n=11 cases) were excluded from this study. The age ranged from 39 to 78 (mean:

59.6±9.3) years old. Overall, 73 patients (20.3%) had Canadian Cardiovascular Society angina class IV symptoms. The preoperative demographic characteristics and risk factors of the two groups of patients are presented in Table 1.

The local ethics committee at Anzhen Hospital & Beijing Institute of Heart, Lung and Blood Vessel Diseases approved the use of clinical data for this study. Written informed consent was obtained from each patient for the surgical or interventional procedure.

**Table 1. Preoperative Baseline Demographic Variables and Risk Factors in the PCI and CABG Groups**

| Patient Demographics and Preoperative Risk Factors | PCI Group (n=232) | CABG Group (n=127) | $P$ (t or $\chi^2$) |
|---|---|---|---|
| Age, yrs | 63.76±8.51 | 61.40±8.13 | 0.011 (2.552) |
| Age older than 65, % | 48.71 | 40.16 | 0.120 (2.418) |
| Female, % | 35.78 | 34.64 | 0.830 (0.046) |
| All type Diabetes mellitus , % | 55.60 | 50.39 | 0.344 (0.896) |
| Insulin-dependent DM,% | 16.38 | 12.60 | 0.338 (0.918) |
| HSCRP(mg/L) | 4.8±1.9 | 4.1±2.1 | 0.002 (3.1214) |
| Hyperlipidemia, % | 79.74 | 77.17 | 0.568 (0.326) |
| Current smoker, % | 56.47 | 57.48 | 0.853 (0.034) |
| Renal insufficiency, % | 7.76 | 7.09 | 0.817 (0.053) |
| Hypertension, % | 69.83 | 66.93 | 0.571 (0.321) |
| Family history of CAD, | 34.05 | 38.58 | 0.392 (0.734) |
| Previous MI, % | 45.29 | 51.18 | 0.283 (1.155) |
| Peripheral vascular disease, % | 8.19 | 7.87 | 0.916 (0.011) |
| EF<35 % | 14.22 | 9.45 | 0.191 (1.707) |
| EF,% | 51.5±17.2 | 53.2±18.9 | 0.388 (0.8643) |
| Congestive heart failure, % | 14.66 | 12.60 | 0.917 (0.011) |
| Transient ischemic attack, % | 2.81 | 3.15 | 0.945 (0.005) |
| Stroke, % | 4.74 | 5.51 | 0.749 (0.102) |
| Pulmonary disease, % | 12.93 | 11.81 | 0.759 (0.094) |
| Pre procedure IABP | 7.5 | 14.17 | 0.0367 (4.371) |
| Aspirin, % | 92.67 | 92.13 | 0.851 (0.035) |
| β-Blocker, % | 78.45 | 81.10 | 0.552 (0.353) |
| CCB, % | 37.93 | 40.16 | 0.679 (0.171) |
| Nitrates, % | 69.40 | 72.44 | 0.772 (0.084) |
| Statins, % | 41.81 | 39.37 | 0.653 (0.02) |
| EKG Diagnosis | | | |
| Sinus rhythm,% | 92.67 | 93.70 | 0.714(0.134) |

| Patient Demographics and Preoperative Risk Factors | PCI Group (n=232) | CABG Group (n=127) | $P$ (t or $\chi^2$) |
|---|---|---|---|
| Atrial fibrillation,% | 6.47 | 4.72 | 0.502(0.452) |
| Other rhythm,% | 0.862 | 1.57 | 0.539(0.378) |
| Enrollment diagnosis, % | | | |
| Silent ischemia,% | 3.45 | 4.72 | 0.550 (0.357) |
| Stable angina,% | 33.19 | 22.04 | 0.027 (4.924) |
| Unstable angina,% | 53.88 | 66.14 | 0.024 (5.073) |
| Acute Myocardium infarction,% | 9.48 | 7.1 | 0.440 (0.597) |
| Diseased vessels, n | | | |
| Single ORCS lesion, % | 6.03 | 0.787 | 0.018 (5.644) |
| ORCS+1 vessel stenosis,% | 30.17 | 11.2 | 0.000 (16.790) |
| ORCS+2 vessel stenosis,% | 34.91 | 36.22 | 0.805 (0.061) |
| ORCS+3 vessel stenosis,% | 28.89 | 51.79 | 0.000 (18.76) |
| Vessel territory with stenosis, % | | | |
| RCA | 100 | 100 | 1 |
| LAD | 64.22 | 78.74 | 0.004 (8,137) |
| LCX | 62.93 | 74.80 | 0.022 (5.243) |
| LMCA | 1.29 | 1.58 | 0.828 (0.047) |
| ORCS with proximal atrial artery (%) | 4.31 | 11.81 | 0.008 (7,127) |
| ORCS with more than 2 vessel lesion (%) | 63.79 | 88.19 | 0.000 (24.457) |
| ORCS with more than 4 lesion | 42.67 | 75.59 | 0.000 (37.150) |
| NO. of segments with stenosis>50%of luminal diameter | | | |
| median | 3 | 4 | |
| IQR | 2-4 | 2-5 | |
| Range | 2-5 | 2-7 | |
| OCRS with CTO lesion | 15.08 | 26.77 | 0.007 (7.218) |
| Calcified OCRS | 9.5 | 21.26 | 0.002 (9.658) |
| Long and tortured OCRS | 7.76 | 18.90 | 0.002 (9.858) |
| >95% stenosis of OCRS | 46.98 | 75.59 | 0.000 (27.421) |
| LV aneurysm | 11.64 | 19.68 | 0.038 (4.291) |

IQR: interquartile range; PTCA: Percutaneous transluminal coronary angioplasty; HSCRP: High-sensitive C-reactive protein; LMCA: left main coronary artery; LAD: left anterior descending artery; LCX: left circumflex artery; RCA: right coronary artery; CAD: coronary artery disease; Value are means±SD when appropriate; stable angina was defined according to Canadian Cardiovascular Society system; unstable angina was classified according to the Braunwald classification. CCB: calcium channel blocker; CTO: chronic total occlusion lesion; EF: ejection fraction; IABP: intraaortic balloon pump.

## Procedure Techniques

PCI was performed under local anesthesia. Two types of commercially available DES (sirolimus-eluting stent and paclitaxel-eluting stent) were used, and stent implantation was performed with standard techniques.

All stents were deployed by high-pressure balloon inflation (>14 atmospheres). The stent implantation strategy for bifurcation lesions, lesions with fresh thrombi, calcification, diffuse disease, or complex anatomical features was at the surgeon's discretion. Complete revascularization was recommended for all diseased arteries with stenosis of ≥50%. Overall, 186 consecutive patients with ORCS received a sirolimus-eluting stent and 46 consecutive patients received a paclitaxel-eluting stent. Coronary stent implantation was performed by 12 principle surgeons affiliated to Anzhen Hospital.

The indications were according to what the surgeon deemed appropriate at the time. The surgeons were not given a strict protocol on how or which intervention should be performed, or the type and number of stents deployed. Direct stenting was performed whenever possible. Routine intravascular ultrasound was deemed unnecessary, unless there was a specific indication. Balloon pre-dilatation was performed, followed by stent implantation using the conventional technique for most patients. Post dilatation was only performed if the primary angiographic result was not satisfactory. Staged PCI was performed in some patients, taking into account vessel size, contrast load and the patient's status.

Antiplatelet therapy with aspirin and clopidogrel (75 mg/day) was started at least 3 days before PCI. In case of an emergency, a loading dose of clopidogrel (300 mg) was given at least 2 hours before the intervention. Unfractionated heparin (70–100 IU/kg) was administered as a bolus dose and followed by intravenous infusion, if necessary, to maintain ACT at >250 seconds. Glycoprotein IIb/IIIa inhibitors were used at the surgeon's discretion. Clopidogrel (75 mg daily) was used for at least 12 months, unless contraindicated.

CABG was performed via a median sternotomy approach under general anesthesia and all isolated CABG was performed with an off-pump procedure. All CABG procedures were performed by six principle surgeons affiliated to Anzhen Hospital. All patients in the CABG Group were advised to continue lifelong aspirin therapy (100 mg daily).

## Study Endpoints

The primary endpoint was the incidence of MACCE within 30 days after the revascularization procedure and during the whole follow-up period. MACCEs were defined as all-cause death, nonfatal myocardial infarction, stroke and repeated revascularization. Repeated revascularization was defined as any PCI or bypass surgery after the first revascularization procedure. Non-Q-wave myocardial infarction was diagnosed according to World Health Organization criteria, including an increase in total creatine kinase (CK) level to $\geq 2\times$ the upper limit of the normal range and an elevated MB isoform level without development of new pathological Q waves. A Q-wave myocardial infarction was present when, in addition to CK elevation, a new pathological Q wave was noted in at least two leads.

## Data Collection

One month after discharge, all surviving patients from both groups were assessed at an outpatient clinic for full review by the cardiac surgeon or cardiologist. New York Heart Association (NYHA) class, troponin (Tn)-I and cardiac enzymes, trans-thoracic echocardiography (TTE) and ECG data were recorded. These variables were evaluated at 3-month intervals at the patient's local cardiac center.

Long-term clinical outcomes were assessed up to December 2008 by reviewing the medical files of their cardiologists or general practitioners, or both, when appropriate. Baseline demographics, procedural data and perioperative outcomes were recorded. For late deaths, the medical files were reviewed by one of the primary investigators of this study. The status of the patients was determined by review of hospital records, follow-up questionnaires, or contact with local physicians at an interval of 3 months after the first outpatient visit. Detailed information, including NYHA functional status, cardiac rhythm, complications and present medications were recorded. At the postoperative follow-up, TTE and ECG were assessed in 346 (97.7%) of the 354 patients surviving hospitalization and the main parameters were collected. Patient demographics, preoperative risk factors and the incidence of adverse postoperative outcomes were retrieved from the Digitalcare database at Anzhen Hospital.

## Table 2. Preoperative Baseline Demographic Variables and Risk Factors of the 105 Propensity-Matched Patients

| Patient Demographics and Preoperative Risk Factors | PCI Group (n=105) | CABG Group (n=105) | $P$ ($\chi^2$) |
|---|---|---|---|
| Age, yrs | 61.56±8.33 | 61.72±8.42 | 0.890 (0.14) |
| Age older than 65, n | 48 | 45 | 0.687 (0.17) |
| Female, n | 37 | 35 | 0.771 (0.09) |
| All type Diabetes mellitus , n | 55 | 52 | 0.679 (0.17) |
| Insulin-dependent DM, n | 17 | 16 | 0.850 (0.04) |
| HSCRP(mg/L) | 4.46±2.15 | 4.51±2.04 | 0.863 (0.17) |
| Hyperlipidemia, n | 80 | 77 | 0.634 (0.23) |
| Current smoker, n | 58 | 55 | 0.678 (0.17) |
| Renal insufficiency, n | 7 | 5 | 0.552 (0.35) |
| Hypertension, n | 70 | 67 | 0.664 (0.19) |
| Family history of CAD, n | 38 | 37 | 0.886 (0.02) |
| Previous MI, n | 51 | 48 | 0.678 (0.17) |
| Peripheral vascular disease, n | 8 | 9 | 0.800 (0.06) |
| EF＜35 % | 15 | 13 | 0.687 (0.17) |
| EF,% | 52.1±17.8 | 52.6±18.5 | 0.842 (0.20) |
| Congestive heart failure, n | 16 | 14 | 0.693 (0.16) |
| Transient ischemic attack, n | 4 | 3 | 0.701 (0.15) |
| Stroke, n | 8 | 7 | 0.789 (0.07) |
| Pulmonary disease, n | 15 | 16 | 0.846 (0.04) |
| Pre procedure IABP | 9 | 8 | 0.800 (0.06) |
| Aspirin, n | 97 | 94 | 0.471 (0.52) |
| β-Blocker, n | 83 | 80 | 0.619 (0.25) |
| CCB, n | 42 | 40 | 0.777 (0.08) |
| Nitrates, n | 68 | 72 | 0.558 (0.34) |
| Statins, n | 42 | 45 | 0.674 (0.18) |
| EKG Diagnosis | | | |
| Sinus rhythm, n | 99 | 101 | 0.752 (0.100) |
| Atrial fibrillation, n | 5 | 4 | 0.733 (0.420) |
| Other rhythm, n | 1 | 0 | 0.303 (0.99) |
| Enrollment diagnosis, | | | |
| Silent ischemia, n | 6 | 4 | 0.517 (0.42) |
| Stable angina, n | 28 | 27 | 0.875 (0.03) |
| Unstable angina, n | 62 | 66 | 0.572 (0.32) |
| Acute myocardium infarction, n | 9 | 8 | 0.800 (0.06) |
| Diseased vessels, n | | | |
| Single ORCS lesion, n | 2 | 3 | 0.651 (0.21) |
| ORCS+1 vessel stenosis, n | 13 | 11 | 0.664 (0.189) |
| ORCS+2 vessel stenosis, n | 37 | 39 | 0.774 (0.08) |
| ORCS+3 vessel stenosis, n | 53 | 52 | 0.890 (0.02) |
| Vessel territory with stenosis | | | |

| Patient Demographics and Preoperative Risk Factors | PCI Group (n=105) | CABG Group (n=105) | $P$ ($\chi^2$) |
|---|---|---|---|
| RCA, n | 105 | 105 | 1.0 (0.00) |
| LAD | 77 | 79 | 0.752 (0.10) |
| LCX | 72 | 75 | 0.651 (0.20) |
| LMCA | 1 | 1 | 1.0 (0.00) |
| ORCS with proximal atrial artery, n | 8 | 9 | 0.800 (0.06) |
| ORCS with more than 2 vessel lesion, n | 84 | 86 | 0.725 (0.12) |
| ORCS with more than 4 lesion | 76 | 78 | 0.755 (0.10) |
| NO. of segments with stenosis>50%of luminal diameter | | | |
| median | 4 | 4 | |
| IQR | 2-4 | 2-4 | |
| Range | 2-5 | 2-5 | |
| OCRS with CTO lesion, n | 19 | 21 | 0.725 (0.12) |
| Calcified OCRS, n | 18 | 19 | 0.856 (0.03) |
| Long and tortured OCRS | 15 | 17 | 0.701 (0.15) |
| >95% stenosis of OCRS | 69 | 72 | 0.659 (0.19) |
| LV aneurysm | 19 | 17 | 0.712 (0.13) |

IQR: interquartile range; PTCA: Percutaneous transluminal coronary angioplasty; HSCRP: High sensitive C-reactive protein; LMCA: left main coronary artery; LAD: left anterior descending artery; LCX: left circumflex artery; RCA: right coronary artery; CAD: coronary artery disease; Value are means±SD when appropriate; stable angina was defined according to Canadian Cardiovascular Society system; unstable angina was classified according to the Braunwald classification. CCB: calcium channel blocker; CTO: chronic total occlusion lesion; EF: ejection fraction; IABP: intraaortic balloon pump.

## Statistical Analysis

All statistical analyses were performed retrospectively with SAS Version 8.2 for Windows (SAS, Cary, NC). Most continuous variables were not normally distributed, as evaluated by Kolmogorov-Smirnov tests. For reasons of uniformity, summary statistics for all continuous variables are presented as medians and 25th and 75th percentiles. Categorical data are summarized as frequencies and percentages. Differences in baseline characteristics between patients undergoing PCI or CABG were analyzed with Wilcoxon rank sum tests, $\chi^2$ tests or Fisher's exact tests, as appropriate. In an attempt to control for selection bias related to the choice of revascularization procedure, propensity scores were estimated using unconditional logistic regression to determine the predicted probability of undergoing CABG relative to PCI for all patients. The variables used in the initial model (38 factors) are shown in Table 2. Patients undergoing CABG (n=127) or PCI (n=232) were then matched 1-to-1 on these variables, with the same propensity score (±0.05), resulting in successful matching of 105 pairs of patients. Variables used to determine the propensity score included an chronic total occlusion (CTO) lesion, ORCS with more than two vessel lesion, ORCS with more than five lesions, severe stenosis >95% in the ORCS, calcified lesion in the ORCS, long and torched lesion, right coronary artery with proximal atrial artery branch, and LV aneurysm. In the matched cohorts, there were no significant differences between the two groups for the preoperative baseline demographic variables and risk factors (Table 2). Kaplan-Meier curves for freedom from MACCE were constructed and the difference between the two groups was compared by a Log-rank test.

# Results

## Revascularization Data

The results are focused on the 105 propensity-matched pairs of patients. The number of revascularized lesions was significantly smaller in the PCI group than in the CABG group. The median number of stents implanted per patient was 3 (3–4), of which 83.26% were sirolimus-eluting stents, and 16.76% were paclitaxel-eluting stents. OPCAB was performed in 100% of patients in the CABG group. The average interval between the diagnostic angiogram and the CABG procedure was 12±6 days. The mean number of anastomoses performed was 3.2 ± 0.9, with 3.1±0.9 conduits. In 90% of the patients, at least one arterial conduit was used, including the LIMA in 95% of the patients, bilateral internal mammary artery in 4% of patients, and radial artery grafts in 5% of the patients. The rate of complete revascularization was significantly higher in the CABG group than in the PCI group.

## Outcomes during the First 30 Days

The mean hospital stay was significantly shorter in the PCI group (4±2 days) than in the CABG group (14 ± 4 days). As shown in Table 3, two patients (1.90%) in the PCI group died because of acute myocardial infarction caused by stent thrombosis (1 patient) and hemorrhage (1 patient).

### Table 3. Clinical End Points Within First 30 days after the revascularization and During Follow-up for the 105 Propensity-Matched Pairs

| MACCE (%) | PCI Group (n=105) | CABG Group (n=105) | OR (95% CI) | $P$ ($\chi^2$) |
|---|---|---|---|---|
| **First 30 days** | | | | |
| No of patients | 105 | 105 | | |
| Death | 2 (1.90%) | 1 (0.95%) | 2.02 (0.18–22.62) | 0.561 (0.34) |
| Myocardium infarction | 3 (2.86%) | 2 (1.90%) | 1.55 (0.25–9.44) | 0.635 (0.23) |
| Stroke | 1 (0.95%) | 3 (0.86%) | 0.33 (0.33–3.19) | 0.313 (1.02) |
| Death/maycardium infarction/stroke | 6 (5.71%) | 6 (5.71%) | 1.0 (0.31–3.21) | 1 (0.00) |
| Redo-CABG | 4 (3.81%) | 0 (0%) | 2.04 (1.78–2.34) | 0.043 (4.08) |
| Redo-PCI | 3 (2.86%) | 1 (0.95%) | 3.06 (0.31–29.89) | 0.313 (1.02) |
| Repeat revascularization | 7 (6.67%) | 1 (0.95%) | 7.43 (0.90–61.48) | 0.65 0.03 (4.68) |
| Any MACCE | 13 (12.38%) | 7 (6.67%) | 1.98 (0.76–5.18) | 0.158 (1.989) |
| **Late follow-up** | | | | |
| No of patients | 103 | 104 | | |
| Death | 5 (4.85%) | 1 (0.96%) | 5.26 (0.60–45.79) | 0.095 (2.79) |
| Myocardium infarction | 10 (9.71%) | 4 (3.85%) | 2.07 (0.82–8.87) | 0.093 (2.82) |
| Stroke | 4 (3.89%) | 5 (4.81%) | 0.80 (0.21–3.06) | 0.744 (0.11) |
| Death/myocardial infarction/stroke | 19 (18.45%) | 10 (9.62%) | 2.13 (0.94–4.83) | 0.067 (3.35) |
| Redo-CABG | 5 (4.85%) | 0 (0%) | 2.06 (1.79–2.38) | 0.023 (5.17) |
| Redo-PCI | 3 (2.91%) | 2 (1.92%) | 1.53 (0.25–9.35) | 0.643 (0.22) |
| Repeat revascularization | 8 (7.77%) | 2 (1.92%) | 4.30 (0.90–20.74) | 0.05 (3.84) |
| Any MACCE | 27 (26.21%) | 12 (11.54%) | 2.57 (1.18–5.57) | 0.0215 (5.96) |

MACCEs: Major Adverse Cardiac and Cerebrovascular events.

Three patients experienced non-fatal Q-wave (1 patient) or non-Q-wave (2 patients) myocardial infarction. One patient suffered a non-fatal stroke. Three patients (2.86%) needed repeat intervention, and four patients needed emergency bypass surgery. The procedural success rate was 93.33%.

In the CABG group, one patient (0.95%) died because of perioperative acute myocardial infarction. Two patients experienced non-fatal Q-wave (1 patient) or non-Q-wave (1 patient) myocardial infarction. Three patients suffered a non-fatal stroke. Acute repeat PCI was required in one patient (0.95%). No patients required emergency bypass surgery. The $\chi^2$ tests revealed that, of all MACCE events reported during the 30-day in-hospital stay, only emergency CABG for the PCI group relative to the CABG group reached statistical significance (odds ratio [OR]: 2.040; 95% confidence interval [CI]: 1.775–2.27, P=0.043, $\chi^2$=4.078).

## Late Clinical Follow-up

Follow-up was completed in 98.06% and 99.04% of patients in the PCI and CABG groups, respectively. With a mean follow-up of 12.04±6.47 months and a total of 210.67 patient–years in the PCI group, five patients (4.85%) died as a result of exacerbated heart failure (1 patient), life-threatening arrhythmia (1 patient), intracranial bleeding (1 patient), and fatal myocardial infarction (2 patients). Ten patients (9.71%) had non-fatal myocardial infarction, with Q-wave myocardial infarction caused by angiographically confirmed late stent thrombosis in four patients and non-Q-wave myocardial infarction in six patients. Four patients (3.89%) suffered non-fatal stroke. Repeat intervention was required in three patients (2.91%), and five patients (4.85%) required bypass surgery.

In the CABG group, only one patient died (0.97%), which was due to heart failure. Four patients (3.88%) experienced non-fatal acute myocardial infarction. Five patients (4.85%) had non-fatal stroke. Repeat PCI was required in two patients (1.94%), with native coronary arteries in one patient and saphenous venous grafts in one patient. No patient underwent repeated bypass surgery.

The χ2 tests revealed that, of all MACCEs recorded in the late follow-up, the likelihood of undergoing bypass surgery (OR: 2.061; 95% CI: 1.788–2.376, P=0.023, $\chi^2$=5.174) and any MACCE (OR: 2.568; 95% CI: 1.184–5.570, P=0.0215, $\chi^2$=5.963) reached statistical significance for PCI relative to CABG. The Kaplan-Meier freedom from MACCE curves for the PCI and

CABG groups are shown in Figure 1. As shown in Table 4, the Log rank test revealed a significant difference in the freedom from MACCE between the two groups ($\chi^2$=4.48, P=0.0348).

# Discussion

Coronary revascularization methods continue to be refined. In previous studies, percutaneous balloon angioplasty alone has been associated with high restenosis rates of up to 60% for non aorto-ostial lesions and 71% for aorto-ostial lesions [4]. The widespread use of coronary stenting has significantly decreased the need for emergency CABG surgery among patients treated with PCI. The recent introduction of DES has further decreased the incidence of coronary restenosis and the need for repeat revascularization [5]. Since the introduction of DES in 2002, randomized trials [6, 7] have consistently demonstrated that DES reduce restenosis compared with bare metal stents (BMS) in patients with single lesions. Furthermore, single-center registries [8,9,10] have also reported the efficacy of DES for multi-vessel disease. The first major trial in the DES era for the treatment of multi-vessel disease was the ARTS II trial [11], which enrolled 607 patients with MVD treated with sirolimus-eluting stents. The findings of the ARTS II trial were compared with those of the earlier, randomized ARTS trial in which 605 patients underwent bypass surgery and 600 patients received a BMS (n = 600). Although more patients enrolled in the ARTS-II trial had diabetes or more complex lesions, the rate of major cardiovascular events at 1 year was similar between the ARTS II (treated with DES) and CABG treatment in the ARTS trial (10.4% vs. 11.6%, respectively). These findings indicate that the use of DES may offer a promising alternative to CABG in the treatment of patients with MVD. Because restenosis was the principle factor prompting surgery in the earlier randomized clinical trials that compared PCI with CABG, DES may reduce restenosis to reduce the rate of restenisis to <10% in relatively simple cases. Thus, many cardiologists may believe that PCI with DES is at least equivalent, if not superior, to bypass surgery.

Percutaneous treatment of stenosis involving aorto-ostial lesions is technically demanding and has been associated with lower procedural success and worse clinical and angiographic outcomes when compared with non-ostial lesions [12]. Pathophysiologically, the presence of an ostial lesion poses a special management problem for PCI because ostial lesions are more likely to be associated with suboptimal angiographic results as a result of lesion rigidity and recoil[13]. As a special entity of aorto-ostial lesion, ORCS should be emphasized in the treatment of the coronary artery disease. However, the impact of DES on the clinical outcomes of patients with ORCS have yet to be determined. Although stents provide adequate scaffolding to prevent recoil, the rate of in-stent restenosis is still relatively high [14]. Earlier studies that used a BMS showed that restenosis rates are higher for ostial lesions than non-ostial lesions [15]. Furthermore, chronic stent recoil, accounting in part for stent restenosis, occurred only at the junction of the right coronary artery (RCA) and the aortic wall. Utilization of DES in this complex lesion subset is feasible and associated with favorable angiographic results at 7 months; however, the gradual increase in later events at up to 2 years suggests that aorto-ostial disease remains problematic, even in the DES era [16].These findings may be related to the distinctive anatomic structure and geometric characteristics of the RCA ostium. The RCA ostium is pathologically reported to be rich in fibro-cellular tissue and dense adventitia [17]. In-stent restenosis tends to occur in areas of stent recoil. Mechanical forces, such as the lack of arterial distensibility and excessive rigidity, appear to be key factors in causing restenosis at this particular location.

Rocha-Singh et al. [18]reported excellent initial and intermediate outcomes of aorto-ostial stenting (including vein graft anastomosis) with procedural success and overall restenosis rats of 93% and 28%, respectively, at the angiographic follow-up at 5.8 months. On the other hand, other investigators have reported that lesion complexity impedes optimal stent deployment, resulting in a comparatively high prevalence of restenosis and revascularization, particularly in RCA aorto-ostial stenosis [19,20]. Restenosis in the aorto-ostial location is extremely serious because a large myocardial territory is at risk [21].

The SYNTAX (Synergy Between Percutaneous Coronary Intervention With TAXUS and Cardiac Surgery) study [22], which compared PCI with DES versus CABG, revealed that A SYNTAX score threshold of 34 may identify patients who would benefit most from surgical revascularization in terms of reducing risk of mortality. The SYNTAX study provided a deep insight into left main lesion and/or three vessel lesions, but it did not provide interventional guidance for specific lesions, such as ORCS. Our retrospective study included patients with ORCS lesions and expands on the findings of the SYNTAX study.

The efficacy of the off-pump technique in ostial patients is also unknown. In the DES era, which technique is superior for ORCS lesions, CABG or PCI?

To address this question, the present study compared the early and mid-term clinical outcomes of off-pump CABG and PCI in ORCS patients. PCI was only performed using DES, and most of the CABG procedures were performed with ITA grafting and SV. Our study, by reviewing 105 propensity score-matched pairs of patients, revealed a benefit in terms of fewer instances of repeat revascularization with the CABG procedure versus the PCI procedure in patients with ORCS during first 30 days and the later follow-up period. The MACCE-free survival rate was also significantly higher in the CABG group than in the PCI group.

To our knowledge, our study is the first to compare the clinical outcomes of PCI using DES versus off-pump CABG in patients with ORCS lesions in the real world. However, what is the optimal management of OCRS lesions? Our analysis revealed that, despite the improved durability of contemporary PCI with DES, the long-term MACCE-free survival rates do not seem to have improved in a similar manner. Because of this risk profile, which is most often associated with ORCS, CABG was regarded as the preferred revascularization method because of its ability to bypass the excess plaque burden and to improve the complete revascularization rates and thus reduce the need for repeat revascularizations.

### Table 4. Freedom from MACCEs in the PCI and CABG Group for 105 Propensity matched Pairs (%)

|            | PCI Group   | CABG Group  | P* value($\chi^2$) |
|------------|-------------|-------------|--------------------|
| 6 months   | 92.74±2.65  | 96.81±1.82  | 0.035 (4.48)       |
| 12 months  | 79.93±4.42  | 92.11±3.17  |                    |
| 18 months  | 65.34±6.31  | 82.80±5.29  |                    |

* Log-rank test for Kaplan-Meier MACCE-free curve between the PCI and CABG groups.

Most cardiac events in the PCI group were attributed to dissection of the right ostial lesions or restenosis of the target vessels. Meanwhile, the good clinical outcomes in the CABG group were attributed to the high patency rate of the bypass graft, particularly with LIMA graft. Furthermore, PCI with multiple stents has an inherent limitation compared with CABG because PCI usually only treats the focal area corresponding to significant stenosis while CABG may bypass the vulnerable plaques that could potentially develop into notable lesions over time. Why is PCI of ostial lesions still associated with adverse outcomes in the DES era? First, the location of the ostial lesion may be a marker for more extensive and advanced atherosclerosis. Second, there are a number of technical factors that may play a role in the relatively poor outcomes of ostial PCI. Indeed, accurate stent placement may be challenging, while elastic recoil and restenosis may occur if the lesion is not completely covered by a stent at its proximal end. This is a particular problem with aorto-ostial (RCA) lesions. Other factors include the vessel angulation, the ability for adequate guide support and adequate stent expansion.

## Study Limitations

This study is a retrospective analysis and some confounding factors may hide any clear association between the early and late prognoses of CABG versus PCI with DES. Although we used propensity score analysis to balance the two non-equivalent groups and reduce any bias for a specific revascularization procedure, a prospective randomized study is needed to confirm the findings of this study.

## Conclusion

OCRS lesions pose a special problem for PCI procedures because the outcomes may be poor due to lesion rigidity and elastic recoil. Although DES represents a major breakthrough in reducing restenosis after PCI, for OCRS lesions, CABG may provide some protection over PCI in terms of the freedom from MACCE. This was mainly due to the reduced number of repeat revascularization procedures. Although the difference with CABG surgery has narrowed in the era of stenting, the rate of repeat revascularization procedures remains high after PCI. Therefore, when revascularization is needed for OCRS lesions, Taken together, OCRS lesions are predictive of worse outcomes of PCI and, consequently, CABG should be considered as the first-choice revascularization strategy.

## References

[1]     Tsagalou E, Stancovic G, Ikaovou I, Melzi G, Cosgrave J , Ge L, Michev I, Chieffo A, Airoldi F, Carlino M, Montorfano M, Colombo A.

Early outcome of treatment of ostial de novo left anterior descending coronary artery lesions with drug-eluting stents. *Am J Cardiol* 2006; 97: 187–191.

[2]    Mercado N, Wijns W, Serruys PW, Sigwart U, Flather MD, Stables RH, O'Neill WW, Rodriguez A, Lemos PA, Hueb WA, Gersh BJ, Booth J, Boersma E. One-year outcomes of coronary artery bypass graft surgery versus percutaneous coronary intervention with multiple stenting for multisystem disease: a meta-analysis of individual patient data from randomized clinical trials. *J Thorac Cardiovasc Surg.* 2005 Aug;130(2):512-9.

[3]    Klein LW. Are drug-eluting stents the preferred treatment for multivessel coronary artery disease? *J Am Coll Cardiol* 2006;47:22–26.

[4]    Tan KH, Sulke N, Taub N, Sowton E. Percutaneous transluminal coronary angioplasty of aorta ostial, nonaorta ostial, and branch ostial stenoses: Acute and long-term outcome. *Eur Heart J* 1995;16:631–639.

[5]    Morice MC, Serruys PW, Sousa JE , Fajadet J, Ban Hayashi E, Perin M, Colombo A, Schuler G, Barragan P, Guagliumi G, Molnàr F, Falotico R; RAVEL Study Group. A randomized comparison of a sirolimus-eluting stent with a standard stent for coronary revascularization. *N Engl J Med.* 2002;346:1773-80.

[6]    Moses JW, Leon MB, Popma JJ, Fitzgerald PJ, Holmes DR, O'Shaughnessy C, Caputo RP, Kereiakes DJ, Williams DO, Teirstein PS, Jaeger JL, Kuntz RE; SIRIUS Investigators. Sirolimus-eluting stents versus standard stents in patients with stenosis in a native coronary artery. *N Engl J Med* 2003;349:1315–1323.

[7]    Stone GW, Ellis SG, Cox DA, Hermiller J, O'Shaughnessy C, Mann JT, Turco M, Caputo R, Bergin P, Greenberg J, Popma JJ, Russell ME; TAXUS-IV Investigators. A polymer-based, paclitaxel-eluting stent in patients with coronary artery disease. *N Engl J Med* 2004;250:221–231.

[8]    ampatzis CA, Hoye A, Lemos PA, Saia F, Tanabe K, Degertekin M, Sianos G, Smits PC, van der Giessen WJ, McFadden E, van Domburg R, de Feyter P, Serruys PW. Elective sirolimus-eluting stent implantation for multivessel disease involving significant LAD stenosis: one-year clinical outcomes of 99 consecutive patients--the Rotterdam experience. *Catheter Cardiovasc Interv* 2004;63:57–60.

[9]    Lemos PA, Serruys PW, van Domburg RT, Saia F, Arampatzis CA, Hoye A, Degertekin M, Tanabe K, Daemen J, Liu TK, McFadden E, Sianos G, Hofma SH, Smits PC, van der Giessen WJ, de Feyter PJ. Unrestricted utilization of sirolimus-eluting stents compared with

conventional bare stent implantation in the "real world": The Rapamycin-Eluting Stent Evaluated At Rotterdam Cardiology Hospital (RESEARCH) Registry. *Circulation* 2004;109:190– 195.

[10] Ong AT, Serruys PW, Aoki J, Hoye A, van Mieghem CA, Rodriguez-Granillo GA, Valgimigli M, Sonnenschein K, Regar E, van der Ent M, de Jaegere PP, McFadden EP, Sianos G, van der Giessen WJ, de Feyter PJ, van Domburg RT. The unrestricted use of paclitaxel versus sirolimus-eluting stents for coronary artery disease in an unselected population—One Year Results of The Taxus-Stent Evaluated At Rotterdam Cardiology Hospital (T-SEARCH) Registry. *J Am Coll Cardiol* 2005;45:1135–1141.

[11] Serruys PW. ARTS II. Arterial Revascularization Therapies Study part II of the sirolimus-eluting stent in the treatment of patients with multivessel de novo coronary artery lesions. *EuroInterv* 2005;1:147– 156.

[12] Clin K. An approach to ostial lesion management. *Curr Interv Cardiol Rep* 2001; 3:87–89.

[13] Asakura Y, Takagi S, Ishikawa S, Asakura K, Sueyoshi K, Sakamoto M, et al. Favorable strategy for the ostial lesion of the left anterior descending coronary artery: influence on narrowing of circumflex coronary artery. *Catheter Cardiovasc Diagn* 1998; 43:95–100.

[14] Park SJ, Lee CW, Hong MK, Kim JJ, Park SW. Stent placement for ostial left anterior descending coronary artery stenosis: acute and long-term (2-year) results. *Catheter Cardiovasc Interv* 2000; 49:267–271.

[15] Airoldi F, Di Mario C, Stankovic G, Briguori C, Carlino M, Chieffo A, Liistro F, Montorfano M, Pagnotta P, Spanos V, Tavano D, Colombo A. Clinical and angiographic outcome of directional atherectomy followed by stent implantation in de novo lesions located at the ostium of the left anterior descending coronary artery. *Heart* 2003; 89:1050–1054.

[16] Tsuchida K, Daemen J, Tanimoto S, García-García HM, Kukreja N, Vaina S, Ong AT, Sianos G, de Jaegere PP, van Domburg RT, Serruys PW. Two-year outcome of the use of paclitaxel-eluting stents in aorto-ostial lesions. *Int J Cardiol.* 2007 Nov 19. [Epub ahead of print]

[17] Hong MK, Haudenschild CC, Tjurmin A, Kent KM, Leon MB. Why do aortoostial lesions behave differently than non-ostial lesions? Histologic findings in directional atherectomy specimens of aorto-ostial vs. non-ostial lesions. *J Am Coll Cardiol* 1995; 25:138A.

[18] Rocha-Singh K, Morris N, Wong C, Schatz RA, Teirstein PS. Coronary stenting for treatment of ostial stenoses of native coronary arteries or aortocoronary saphenous venous grafts. Am J Cardiol 1995; 75:26–29.

[19] Zampieri P, Colombo A, Almagor Y, Maiello L, Finci L. Results of coronary stenting of ostial lesions. *Am J Cardiol* 1994; 73:901–903.

[20] Jain SP, Liu MW, Dean LS, Babu R, Goods CM, Yadav JS, Al-Shaibi KF, Mathur A, Iyer SS, Parks JM, Baxley WA, Roubin GS. Comparison of balloon angioplasty versus debulking devices versus stenting in right coronary ostial lesions. *Am J Cardiol* 1997; 79:1334–1338.

[21] Rissanen V. Occurrence of coronary ostial stenosis in a necropsy series of myocardial infarction, sudden death, and violent death. *Br Heart J* 1975; 37:182–191.

[22] Usefulness of SYNTAX score to select patients with left main coronary artery disease to be treated with coronary artery bypass graft. Capodanno D, Capranzano P, Di Salvo ME, Caggegi A, Tomasello D, Cincotta G, Miano M, Patané M, Tamburino C, Tolaro S, Patané L, Calafiore AM, Tamburino C. *JACC Cardiovasc Interv.* 2009 Aug;2(8):731-8.

# Index

**N**

**O**

**P**